BIOHACKING FOR BEGINNERS

Your Journey to a Healthier Life

Kiet Huynh

Table of Contents

PART I
Introduction to Biohacking

Chapter 1: Exploring Biohacking: Understanding the Concept and Benefits

What is Biohacking?

In our fast-paced and ever-evolving world, the quest for better health, enhanced performance, and increased longevity has never been more compelling. The concept of biohacking has emerged as a powerful and revolutionary approach to achieving these goals. But what exactly is biohacking, and what benefits does it offer?

Biohacking is the art and science of optimizing your own biology to reach your full potential. It involves making informed, personalized choices about your lifestyle, nutrition, exercise, and even the use of technology to improve your physical and mental well-being. This book is your guide to understanding the fundamental principles of biohacking and how to apply them to your own life.

In this first chapter, we will delve into the core concept of biohacking, breaking down its components and exploring the myriad benefits it has to offer. From boosting your cognitive performance to enhancing your physical fitness, biohacking holds the promise of a better, healthier, and more empowered you.

But biohacking is not without its ethical considerations and safety concerns. As we embark on this journey of self-improvement, it's vital to be aware of the potential pitfalls and challenges that may arise. Before we explore the exciting world of biohacking in depth, let's begin by gaining a firm grasp of the concept and the incredible benefits it can bring into our lives.

The Benefits of Biohacking

Biohacking, as we have come to understand, is a fascinating journey of self-improvement and optimization. It offers a wide array of benefits, encompassing various aspects of our lives. Here, we'll explore the remarkable advantages of embracing the world of biohacking.

1. Enhanced Physical Performance: Biohacking techniques allow you to push the boundaries of your physical capabilities. Whether your goal is to build strength, increase endurance, or achieve peak athletic performance, biohacking strategies can help you achieve new heights.

2. Improved Cognitive Function: Sharpening your mind and enhancing cognitive function is another significant benefit of biohacking. By fine-tuning your diet, lifestyle, and mental practices, you can boost memory, focus, and overall mental clarity.

3. Increased Energy and Vitality: With biohacking, you can unlock newfound levels of energy and vitality. Say goodbye to mid-afternoon slumps and welcome sustained energy throughout the day.

4. Better Sleep Quality: Quality sleep is the cornerstone of good health. Biohacking provides strategies for improving sleep patterns, ensuring you wake up refreshed and rejuvenated.

5. Longevity and Quality of Life: One of the most compelling aspects of biohacking is its potential to extend your lifespan and improve the quality of your years. By making informed choices, you can increase your chances of living a longer, healthier life.

6. Personal Empowerment: Biohacking puts you in control of your health and well-being. It empowers you to make informed decisions about your body and mind, leading to a greater sense of control over your life.

7. Flexibility and Adaptability: Biohacking is highly adaptable to individual goals and needs. Whether you're seeking weight loss, muscle gain, or mental clarity, you can customize your biohacking journey to fit your unique aspirations.

As we embark on this exploration of biohacking, keep in mind that these benefits are within reach. The subsequent chapters of this book will delve deeper into the strategies and techniques to help you unlock the full potential of biohacking and experience these advantages for yourself.

The Science Behind Biohacking

Biohacking is not merely a collection of wellness trends or self-improvement fads. It is firmly rooted in science, drawing from various fields to help us understand and optimize our own biology. In this section, we will explore the scientific foundations that underpin the art of biohacking.

Biology and Physiology: At the core of biohacking is a deep understanding of human biology and physiology. This includes the intricate workings of our organs, systems, and cells. By comprehending the biological mechanisms that govern our bodies, we can identify areas for improvement and implement targeted interventions.

Genetics: Genetics plays a pivotal role in biohacking. Our genes influence our susceptibility to certain health conditions, our response to different diets, and even our athletic potential. Genetic testing and personalized genetic data are valuable tools in tailoring biohacking strategies to individual needs.

Nutrition and Metabolism: Nutrition is a central pillar of biohacking. Understanding how different nutrients affect our metabolism, energy levels, and overall health is essential. Biohackers often adopt specific diets and dietary interventions based on scientific principles to optimize their well-being.

Neurology and Cognitive Science: For those seeking to enhance mental clarity and cognitive performance, biohacking leverages insights from neurology and cognitive science. Techniques such as mindfulness, nootropics, and brain-training exercises are informed by these fields.

Endocrinology and Hormones: Hormones play a significant role in regulating various bodily functions. Biohacking strategies can influence hormone levels to achieve specific health and performance goals, such as muscle growth or fat loss.

Exercise Physiology: Exercise is a cornerstone of biohacking for physical improvement. Biohackers draw from exercise physiology to design workout routines that optimize results while minimizing the risk of injury.

Technology and Data Analysis: Biohacking often incorporates the latest technological advancements. Wearable devices, apps, and data analysis tools provide biohackers with real-time data on their health and performance, allowing for precise adjustments to their strategies.

The science behind biohacking is a dynamic and evolving field, with ongoing research and discoveries. As we dive deeper into this book, we will explore how to apply this scientific knowledge to create personalized biohacking plans that can transform your health and well-being.

Ethical Considerations and Safety

As we embark on our journey to explore the fascinating world of biohacking, it is essential to consider the ethical dimensions and safety aspects associated with this practice. Biohacking, by its nature, involves actively and intentionally modifying one's biology and lifestyle. Here, we delve into the critical ethical considerations and safety guidelines to ensure that your biohacking journey is both responsible and rewarding.

Ethical Considerations:

1. Informed Consent: When embarking on biohacking experiments or interventions, it is crucial to have a full understanding of the potential risks and benefits. Always make informed choices, and, if necessary, consult with healthcare professionals or experts.

2. Privacy: The use of personal data, especially in genetic testing and health monitoring, raises privacy concerns. Be mindful of how your data is collected, stored, and used, and choose trustworthy providers who prioritize data security.

3. Transparency: Be transparent about your biohacking activities, especially if they involve unconventional or experimental approaches. This can help create a culture of openness and shared learning within the biohacking community.

4. Do No Harm: A fundamental ethical principle in biohacking is the commitment to "do no harm." Always prioritize safety and well-being over potentially risky or extreme interventions.

Safety Guidelines:

1. Consultation: Before making significant changes to your lifestyle or health routine, it's advisable to consult with a healthcare professional. They can offer valuable insights and help you make informed decisions.

2. Gradual Progress: Avoid making drastic changes to your diet, exercise, or lifestyle all at once. Gradual adjustments allow your body to adapt and reduce the risk of adverse effects.

3. Monitoring: Regularly monitor your health, especially when experimenting with new biohacking techniques. This includes tracking vital signs, blood markers, and other relevant data.

4. Balanced Approach: Biohacking should promote overall well-being. Avoid becoming fixated on a single aspect of your health at the expense of others. A balanced approach is key.

5. Legal and Regulatory Compliance: Be aware of the legal and regulatory aspects of biohacking in your region. Some biohacking practices may be subject to specific laws or regulations.

6. Community Support: Engage with the biohacking community, both online and offline, to share experiences, learn from others, and receive support. This sense of community can be invaluable in your journey.

Remember, biohacking is a tool for self-improvement and optimization, but it should always be pursued with responsibility and a commitment to ethical conduct and safety. As we progress through this book, we will continue to explore how to navigate these ethical and safety considerations while achieving your biohacking goals.

Chapter 2: Fundamental Principles of the Body's Systems and How They Work

The Human Body: A Complex Network of Systems

The human body is a marvel of complexity and coordination, comprised of a multitude of systems working in harmony to sustain life and maintain optimal function. Understanding the fundamental principles of these systems is a vital step in the journey of biohacking.

Systems of the Human Body:

Our bodies consist of various interconnected systems, each with a unique set of functions. Some of the primary systems include:

- **Circulatory System:** Responsible for the circulation of blood and oxygen throughout the body.

- **Respiratory System:** Manages the intake of oxygen and removal of carbon dioxide.

- **Digestive System:** Processes and extracts nutrients from the food we consume.

- **Nervous System:** Controls communication between different parts of the body through electrical impulses.

- **Endocrine System:** Regulates hormones, which influence various bodily functions.

- **Muscular System:** Enables movement and supports body structure.

- **Skeletal System:** Provides structural support and protection for vital organs.

- **Immune System:** Defends the body against pathogens and diseases.

- **Lymphatic System:** Maintains fluid balance and supports immune function.

- **Reproductive System:** Manages the perpetuation of our species.

- **Urinary System:** Removes waste products and maintains electrolyte balance.

Homeostasis: The Body's Balancing Act:

One of the critical principles governing the human body is homeostasis. Homeostasis refers to the body's ability to maintain a stable and balanced internal environment despite external changes. It involves the regulation of factors such as temperature, pH, and the concentration of various substances within narrow limits.

Integration of Systems:

The human body is not a collection of isolated systems but a highly integrated network. For instance, the circulatory system provides a means for hormones produced by the endocrine system to reach their target tissues. The nervous system coordinates the actions of different body parts. Understanding these interconnections is essential for effective biohacking.

Individual Variation:

It's crucial to recognize that individuals can exhibit significant variation in how their body systems function. Genetic, environmental, and lifestyle factors all play a role in these differences. Biohacking embraces this individuality and tailors strategies to meet specific needs and goals.

As we delve deeper into the world of biohacking, this foundational knowledge of the human body's systems and their interplay will provide the basis for making informed decisions about optimizing our biology. We will explore how to leverage this understanding to enhance various aspects of health and performance in the chapters that follow.

Homeostasis: The Body's Balancing Act

The human body is a remarkable self-regulating system, constantly striving to maintain a state of equilibrium known as homeostasis. Homeostasis is the body's innate ability to keep its internal environment stable, even in the face of external changes and challenges. This concept is central to understanding the fundamental principles of our body's systems and how they work.

Key Aspects of Homeostasis:

1. Temperature Regulation: The body carefully maintains its core temperature around 98.6°F (37°C). In response to external temperature variations, the body either produces heat or dissipates it to keep temperature within this narrow range.

2. Blood Pressure Control: The circulatory system regulates blood pressure to ensure a consistent flow of oxygen and nutrients to cells throughout the body. Specialized sensors monitor blood pressure and adjust it as needed.

3. Blood Glucose Balance: The body tightly controls blood glucose levels. The pancreas, for example, releases insulin to lower blood sugar levels after a meal and glucagon to raise them when needed.

4. pH Regulation: The body carefully maintains its pH, which is a measure of acidity or alkalinity. Systems such as the respiratory system and the kidneys work together to keep pH within a specific range to support essential chemical reactions.

5. Electrolyte Balance: Homeostasis extends to the regulation of electrolytes, including sodium, potassium, calcium, and others. Proper electrolyte balance is crucial for muscle and nerve function.

6. Fluid Balance: The body maintains an optimal balance of fluids, ensuring that you have enough water and electrolytes to support bodily functions. The kidneys play a vital role in regulating fluid levels.

The Role of Feedback Mechanisms:

Homeostasis relies on feedback mechanisms. When the body detects a deviation from the desired set point, it activates processes to bring the system back into balance. There are two main types of feedback mechanisms:

1. Negative Feedback: This is the most common type of feedback mechanism in homeostasis. It works to counteract any changes from the set point. For example, if body temperature rises, the body sweats to cool down.

2. Positive Feedback: In this type of mechanism, the body reinforces a change from the set point. It is less common in maintaining homeostasis and is often associated with processes like blood clotting and uterine contractions during childbirth.

Understanding the concept of homeostasis is essential for biohackers because many biohacking strategies aim to influence or optimize these systems. By gaining insights into how the body naturally regulates its internal environment, biohackers can make informed choices to promote health, performance, and well-being.

In the following sections of this book, we will explore specific biohacking techniques and interventions that leverage the body's homeostatic mechanisms to achieve desired outcomes.

The Role of Genetics in Biohacking

Genetics, the study of our unique genetic code, plays a pivotal role in the field of biohacking. Your genes are the blueprint that shapes your biology, influencing everything from your physical characteristics to your susceptibility to certain health conditions. Understanding the role of genetics in biohacking is essential to crafting personalized strategies for optimal well-being.

The Human Genome:

The human genome is the complete set of an individual's genetic information. It is composed of DNA, a long, complex molecule that contains the instructions for building and operating the body. The human genome consists of approximately 20,000 to 25,000 protein-coding genes, but it also includes non-coding regions that regulate gene activity.

Genetic Variability:

No two individuals have the exact same genetic makeup, except for identical twins. Genetic variability is responsible for the diversity in traits and susceptibility to different health conditions among people. Variations in genes can influence how our bodies respond to diet, exercise, and various environmental factors.

Personalized Biohacking:

One of the most compelling aspects of genetics in biohacking is the potential for personalization. By analyzing your genetic data, you can gain insights into how your body is wired. This information can guide personalized biohacking strategies, including:

- **Dietary Choices:** Genetic testing can reveal how your body metabolizes certain nutrients and which dietary patterns may be most beneficial for you.

- **Exercise Optimization:** Genetic information can inform your exercise routine, helping you understand your potential for muscle development, endurance, and other athletic traits.

- **Health Risk Assessment:** Genetic tests can identify your predisposition to specific health conditions, allowing you to take proactive steps to mitigate risks.

- **Nutritional Supplementation:** Based on genetic data, you can tailor your supplement choices to address potential deficiencies.

Ethical Considerations:

While genetic information can be a powerful tool for biohacking, it also raises ethical concerns. Protecting the privacy of genetic data and ensuring responsible use of this information is paramount. Ethical considerations in genetic biohacking include informed consent, data security, and the responsible sharing of genetic insights.

As we progress through this book, we will explore how to incorporate genetic information into your biohacking journey. Whether your goal is enhanced performance, better health, or longevity, understanding your genetics can help you unlock the full potential of personalized biohacking.

The Impact of Lifestyle and Environment

While genetics provides a blueprint for your biology, the way you live your life and the environment you inhabit have a profound influence on your health and well-being. This section explores how lifestyle and environmental factors play a significant role in shaping your body's systems and overall biology.

Lifestyle Choices:

Your daily choices, from what you eat to how much you exercise and how well you manage stress, have a substantial impact on your health and performance. Lifestyle biohacking involves optimizing these choices to achieve your desired goals. Some key aspects of lifestyle biohacking include:

- **Diet and Nutrition:** The food you consume provides the building blocks for your body. By making informed dietary choices, you can influence factors like energy levels, weight management, and overall health.

- **Physical Activity:** Regular exercise is a cornerstone of a healthy lifestyle. Biohackers design exercise routines that align with their goals, whether that's building strength, improving endurance, or enhancing mental clarity.

- **Sleep Quality:** Quality sleep is essential for the body's repair and recovery. Lifestyle biohackers prioritize sleep to enhance physical and cognitive performance.

- **Stress Management:** Chronic stress can have a detrimental impact on your health. Biohackers employ stress management techniques, such as meditation and mindfulness, to maintain mental and emotional balance.

Environmental Factors:

Your environment also exerts a significant influence on your biology. Environmental biohacking involves making conscious choices about the spaces you inhabit and the external factors you expose yourself to. Key considerations include:

- **Air Quality:** The quality of the air you breathe can affect your respiratory health. Environmental biohackers might use air purifiers and ensure proper ventilation.

- **Nutrition Access:** The availability of healthy food choices in your environment can impact your dietary decisions. Access to fresh and nutritious options is a priority for many biohackers.

- **Light Exposure:** Light, especially natural sunlight, plays a role in regulating your circadian rhythms. Biohackers may incorporate light exposure strategies to enhance sleep and wake cycles.

- **Chemical Exposure:** Reducing exposure to harmful chemicals and toxins in your environment is essential. This can include choices about the products you use and the quality of your water supply.

- **Geographical Location:** Your geographical location can affect your lifestyle, including the availability of outdoor activities and exposure to different climates.

Understanding the interplay between your lifestyle choices and your environment is vital for biohacking success. By making conscious decisions in these areas, you can create a supportive foundation for your biohacking journey and optimize your biology for improved health, performance, and overall well-being.

As we continue with this book, we will explore specific biohacking strategies that leverage lifestyle and environmental factors to enhance various aspects of your life.

Chapter 3: Why Biohacking Is a Wise Choice for Everyone

The Health Crisis and the Need for Personalized Solutions

In our modern world, health and well-being have become increasingly important and often elusive goals. The prevalence of chronic diseases, the pressures of a sedentary lifestyle, and the challenges posed by environmental factors have collectively created a health crisis. In the face of these issues, the need for personalized solutions has never been more critical. This section delves into the health crisis and the role of personalized biohacking in addressing it.

The Modern Health Crisis:

- **Rising Chronic Diseases:** Chronic diseases, such as heart disease, diabetes, and obesity, are on the rise. These conditions significantly impact the quality of life and place a substantial burden on healthcare systems.

- **Lifestyle-Related Factors:** Sedentary lifestyles, poor dietary choices, and high-stress levels have contributed to the emergence of many health issues. These factors are largely preventable through conscious lifestyle changes.

- **Environmental Challenges:** Environmental factors, including pollution, toxins, and changing climates, can affect health and well-being. These challenges underscore the importance of adapting to an ever-changing world.

The Limitations of One-Size-Fits-All Solutions:

Traditional approaches to health and wellness often provide generic recommendations that may not be effective for everyone. One-size-fits-all solutions fail to consider the individuality of each person's biology, genetics, and lifestyle. This is where biohacking shines, as it embraces the concept of personalized solutions.

The Power of Personalization:

Biohacking empowers individuals to take control of their health and well-being through personalized strategies. By understanding your unique genetic makeup, biology, and lifestyle, you can tailor interventions that address your specific needs and goals. Personalization allows for:

- **Targeted Health Improvement:** Rather than applying broad recommendations, biohacking identifies precise areas for improvement based on individual strengths and weaknesses.

- **Enhanced Performance:** Biohacking strategies can optimize physical and cognitive performance, helping you reach your full potential.

- **Prevention and Longevity:** Personalized biohacking can address health risks early and promote longevity by making proactive choices that suit your biology.

- **Sustainability:** Personalized solutions are more likely to be sustainable because they align with your preferences and needs.

In an era where health challenges are widespread, biohacking offers a path forward that is both practical and effective. By embracing personalized biohacking strategies, individuals can reclaim their health and well-being, address specific concerns, and proactively work towards a brighter, healthier future.

In the subsequent chapters of this book, we will explore the myriad ways in which biohacking can be harnessed to address the unique health and performance goals of individuals.

The Potential for Enhanced Performance

Biohacking is not limited to addressing health concerns alone; it also offers a remarkable potential for enhancing various aspects of performance in our daily lives. In this section, we'll explore how biohacking can elevate your physical and cognitive performance to help you achieve your full potential.

Physical Performance Enhancement:

- **Strength and Endurance:** Biohacking techniques can help you build strength and improve endurance. Whether you're a professional athlete or simply someone seeking to enhance your physical capabilities, biohacking can fine-tune your exercise routines and nutrition for optimal results.

- **Weight Management:** Biohacking strategies can aid in weight management by optimizing your metabolism, dietary choices, and exercise regimens to achieve and maintain a healthy weight.

- **Recovery:** Improved recovery techniques, such as sleep optimization and nutrition, can minimize post-workout fatigue and soreness, allowing you to train more efficiently and consistently.

- **Injury Prevention:** By tailoring exercise routines and addressing individual biomechanical factors, biohacking can reduce the risk of injuries during physical activities.

Cognitive Enhancement:

- **Mental Clarity:** Biohacking practices can enhance mental clarity, focus, and cognitive function. Techniques such as mindfulness meditation and specific dietary choices can boost brain function.

- **Memory and Learning:** Biohacking approaches aim to improve memory retention and accelerate the learning process. Nootropics, cognitive exercises, and brain-training techniques are among the tools at your disposal.

- **Emotional Well-being:** Stress management techniques, combined with personalized approaches to emotional well-being, can help you maintain a positive mental state.

- **Creativity:** Certain biohacking methods have been linked to increased creativity, enabling you to think outside the box and approach problems with innovative solutions.

Lifestyle Optimization:

Biohacking is not limited to physical and mental performance. It also encompasses broader lifestyle optimization. By fine-tuning your daily routines, you can:

- **Boost Productivity:** Increase your productivity and efficiency by optimizing your daily schedule, improving time management, and identifying optimal work-rest cycles.

- **Quality Sleep:** Enjoy higher-quality sleep by addressing sleep-related issues through biohacking. This, in turn, enhances your physical and cognitive performance during the day.

- **Stress Reduction:** Biohacking strategies for stress management can lead to a more relaxed and balanced lifestyle, improving your overall well-being.

- **Longevity:** Some biohacking practices are focused on increasing your chances of living a longer, healthier life by addressing the aging process at the cellular level.

The potential for enhanced performance through biohacking is vast and adaptable to individual goals. Whether you're looking to excel in your career, athletic pursuits, or creative endeavors, biohacking provides a set of tools to help you reach new heights and unlock your full potential.

In the following chapters, we will delve deeper into the specific biohacking techniques that can be employed to optimize physical and cognitive performance and achieve your personal goals.

Longevity and Quality of Life

Longevity, the desire for a long and healthy life, is a common aspiration for many. Biohacking offers a unique approach to not only extending the years you have but also ensuring that those years are filled with vitality, quality, and a high standard of living. In this section, we'll explore how biohacking can contribute to both longevity and the overall quality of life.

Extending Lifespan:

Biohacking strategies aimed at extending lifespan are based on understanding the processes of aging at the cellular and molecular levels. Some of these include:

- **Telomere Lengthening:** Telomeres are protective caps at the ends of chromosomes that naturally shorten with age. Certain biohacking practices aim to slow down or reverse telomere shortening, potentially extending the lifespan of cells.

- **Caloric Restriction:** Controlled caloric restriction is a well-studied method in biohacking that may extend lifespan by promoting metabolic efficiency and reducing the risk of age-related diseases.

- **Nutritional Optimization:** Personalized nutrition plans and specific dietary interventions can influence factors associated with aging, such as inflammation and oxidative stress.

Quality of Life:

Longevity isn't just about living longer; it's also about living better. Biohacking aims to enhance the overall quality of life as you age. This involves strategies for:

- **Maintaining Mobility:** Biohacking can address issues related to muscle loss, joint health, and mobility, helping you stay active and independent.

- **Cognitive Health:** By optimizing cognitive function, biohacking can support memory, mental clarity, and emotional well-being as you age.

- **Energy and Vitality:** Biohacking interventions can help you maintain high energy levels and a youthful vitality throughout your life.

- **Disease Prevention:** A proactive approach to health, including personalized risk assessments and interventions, can reduce the risk of chronic diseases associated with aging.

Healthy Aging:

Biohacking is not about defying the natural aging process, but about aging in a healthier and more graceful manner. Biohackers aim to age with resilience, maintaining their physical and mental well-being as they progress through the years.

Lifestyle and Longevity:

Your lifestyle choices and environment also play significant roles in determining both your lifespan and the quality of those years. Biohacking involves:

- **Stress Reduction:** Strategies for managing and reducing stress, which can have a significant impact on the aging process.

- **Sleep Optimization:** High-quality sleep is crucial for healthy aging. Biohacking practices often focus on improving sleep patterns.

- **Physical Activity:** Regular exercise and movement are cornerstones of healthy aging, and biohacking techniques can optimize your fitness routines.

- **Environmental Adaptation:** Adapting your living environment to support your well-being, including air and water quality, can contribute to healthy aging.

By understanding the principles of biohacking, individuals can take proactive steps to promote longevity and ensure that they not only live longer lives but also enjoy those years to the fullest.

In the upcoming chapters, we will explore specific biohacking techniques and interventions that can be employed to support both longevity and an enhanced quality of life.

Individual Empowerment and Personal Goals

Biohacking is a journey of self-empowerment, where individuals take control of their own biology and well-being. It allows for the pursuit of personal goals, enabling you to customize your path to a healthier, more vibrant life. In this section, we'll explore how biohacking empowers individuals and supports the pursuit of personal aspirations.

Taking Control of Your Health:

Biohacking shifts the responsibility for health and well-being from external sources to the individual. It empowers you to make informed decisions and actively manage your health. This includes:

- **Self-Awareness:** Biohacking encourages self-awareness, helping you better understand your body, its needs, and its unique responses to different interventions.

- **Proactive Health Management:** Rather than waiting for health issues to arise, biohacking is about taking proactive steps to prevent problems and optimize well-being.

- **Personalized Health Plans:** Biohacking allows you to create customized health plans that align with your specific goals and aspirations.

Customized Goals and Outcomes:

One of the strengths of biohacking is its adaptability to individual goals. Whether you seek better physical performance, enhanced mental clarity, improved emotional well-being, or specific health outcomes, biohacking can be tailored to meet your aspirations.

- **Performance Enhancement:** If your goal is to excel in athletics, professional life, or creative endeavors, biohacking strategies can be fine-tuned to support these ambitions.

- **Weight Management:** Whether you aim to lose weight, gain muscle, or maintain a healthy weight, biohacking offers strategies to achieve these goals.

- **Cognitive Enhancement:** For those seeking sharper mental focus, improved memory, or heightened creativity, biohacking provides tools to optimize cognitive function.

- **Emotional Well-being:** Biohacking techniques can support emotional balance and help you navigate life's challenges with resilience and well-being.

Holistic Approach:

Biohacking promotes a holistic approach to well-being, recognizing that health is a multifaceted concept that encompasses physical, mental, and emotional dimensions. This holistic perspective allows for the pursuit of well-rounded personal goals.

Lifelong Learning:

Biohacking is a journey of continuous learning and self-improvement. It encourages individuals to explore new strategies, adapt to changing circumstances, and refine their approaches based on their evolving goals.

Community Support:

Within the biohacking community, individuals find support, share experiences, and learn from one another. This sense of community empowers individuals in their biohacking journey and helps them achieve their personal goals.

Whether your aspirations involve pushing the boundaries of your physical capabilities, enhancing your mental acuity, or simply living a healthier and more fulfilling life, biohacking provides a toolkit for achieving your individual goals. By understanding the principles and practices of biohacking, you can embark on a journey of self-empowerment and personal growth.

The Flexibility of Biohacking

One of the key strengths of biohacking is its remarkable flexibility. Biohacking is not a one-size-fits-all approach but rather a dynamic and adaptable journey. In this section, we'll explore the inherent flexibility of biohacking and how it allows individuals to customize their paths to well-being.

Personalized Approaches:

Biohacking recognizes that each individual is unique, with distinct genetics, biology, goals, and lifestyles. This recognition drives the customization of biohacking strategies to suit individual needs. The flexibility of biohacking enables:

- **Personalized Nutrition:** You can choose dietary approaches that align with your metabolism, preferences, and health goals.

- **Tailored Exercise:** Your exercise routines can be designed to match your fitness objectives, whether that's strength, endurance, or agility.

- **Optimal Sleep Patterns:** Biohacking strategies can be adapted to your sleep patterns and circadian rhythms for maximum rest and recovery.

- **Stress Management:** Techniques for managing stress can be customized to your specific emotional and mental well-being requirements.

Continuous Adaptation:

Biohacking is a journey of constant adaptation. As individuals evolve, their biohacking strategies can evolve with them. This adaptability ensures that biohacking remains relevant and effective throughout life.

- **Changing Goals:** As your goals change over time, biohacking allows you to adapt your strategies to align with these new aspirations.

- **Life Transitions:** Biohacking can accommodate life transitions such as career changes, parenthood, and retirement, ensuring that well-being remains a priority.

- **Aging and Health:** Biohacking can address the evolving health needs and considerations that come with aging.

Combining Approaches:

Biohacking is not confined to a single methodology but instead integrates various approaches to achieve well-being. This integrative approach allows you to combine different biohacking strategies to suit your needs.

- **Diet and Exercise:** The synergy between diet and exercise is just one example of how biohacking combines approaches for optimal results.

- **Mental and Physical Well-being:** Combining strategies for mental clarity and physical performance is common in biohacking.

- **Lifestyle and Environment:** Addressing lifestyle and environmental factors simultaneously allows for a comprehensive approach to well-being.

Data-Driven Decision Making:

The flexibility of biohacking is rooted in data-driven decision making. By monitoring and analyzing data, individuals can adjust their strategies based on real-time information and feedback.

- **Quantified Self:** Many biohackers employ the concept of the "quantified self," using data from wearable devices and health trackers to make informed decisions.

- **Self-Experimentation:** Biohackers often engage in self-experimentation to test the effectiveness of various strategies and adapt accordingly.

Community and Knowledge Sharing:

The biohacking community provides a platform for individuals to share knowledge, experiences, and insights. This collective wisdom fosters flexibility by offering diverse perspectives and approaches.

- **Community Support:** Within the biohacking community, individuals can seek guidance, share successes and challenges, and learn from others' experiences.

- **Continuous Learning:** The dynamic nature of biohacking encourages individuals to engage in continuous learning, staying up-to-date with the latest research and practices.

Biohacking's inherent flexibility empowers individuals to create a journey of well-being that is uniquely tailored to their needs and goals. As you progress through this book, you'll discover a wide array of biohacking techniques and strategies that can be adapted to your individual path to a healthier and more fulfilling life.

PART II
Foundations for Successful Biohacking

Chapter 4: Focus on Lifestyle: How to Prepare Your Body for Biohacking

The Significance of Lifestyle Choices in Biohacking

In the realm of biohacking, lifestyle choices play a pivotal role in shaping the foundation for success. Your daily habits and decisions influence your health, performance, and overall well-being. This section explores the profound significance of lifestyle choices in biohacking and how they set the stage for a successful biohacking journey.

Lifestyle as the Bedrock:

Your lifestyle is the cornerstone upon which the edifice of biohacking is built. It encompasses the choices you make regarding diet, physical activity, sleep, stress management, and more. These choices collectively shape your biological landscape and create the context within which biohacking interventions take place.

The Influence of Lifestyle on Health:

Your lifestyle choices significantly impact your health. Consider the following aspects:

- **Dietary Choices:** What you eat can either fuel your body with essential nutrients or burden it with excessive calories and harmful substances. Diet plays a central role in biohacking for better health.

- **Physical Activity:** The level of physical activity you engage in determines your fitness and, to some extent, your mental health. Exercise is a vital component of a healthy lifestyle.

- **Sleep Quality:** Adequate, high-quality sleep is essential for repair and regeneration. Poor sleep can negatively affect your overall health.

- **Stress Management:** Chronic stress can take a toll on your mental and physical well-being. Lifestyle choices related to stress management can significantly impact your biohacking journey.

The Interplay Between Lifestyle and Genetics:

Lifestyle choices are not isolated from genetics. Your unique genetic makeup interacts with your lifestyle to influence your health and well-being. Biohacking recognizes this interplay and leverages it to create personalized strategies.

- **Nutrigenomics:** The field of nutrigenomics explores how your genetics can inform dietary choices. By understanding your genetic predispositions, you can tailor your diet for optimal health.

- **Exercise Genetics:** Genetic insights can guide your exercise routines, helping you choose activities that align with your body's natural inclinations and strengths.

The Personalization of Biohacking:

Biohacking embraces the idea that one size does not fit all. It's about recognizing that individual bodies respond uniquely to interventions. The significance of lifestyle choices lies in their potential for personalization.

- **Personalized Nutrition:** Dietary choices can be personalized based on your genetics, preferences, and health goals.

- **Optimized Exercise:** Your exercise regimen can be tailored to align with your specific fitness objectives and body type.

- **Lifestyle Factors:** Stress management, sleep patterns, and other lifestyle factors can be adjusted to suit your individual needs.

The Long-Term Impact:

The lifestyle choices you make today can have a lasting impact on your future health and well-being. Biohacking is about creating sustainable, long-term change, and your lifestyle forms the basis for this change.

- **Sustainability:** By making lifestyle choices that are sustainable and enjoyable, you're more likely to maintain these habits over time.

- **Preventive Health:** A healthy lifestyle is one of the most potent tools for preventing chronic diseases and enhancing longevity.

As you embark on your biohacking journey, it's essential to recognize the profound significance of your lifestyle choices. They are the building blocks upon which you will construct your path to better health, enhanced performance, and a more fulfilling life.

In the upcoming sections, we will delve deeper into specific lifestyle choices and biohacking techniques that can prepare your body for a successful biohacking journey.

Dietary Preparation for Biohacking

Diet is a fundamental component of biohacking, and it's where many individuals begin their journey towards better health and well-being. In this section, we'll delve into the importance of dietary preparation for successful biohacking and how the food you consume can serve as a powerful tool in optimizing your body.

Food as Fuel:

The concept of "food as fuel" is a central theme in biohacking. Your dietary choices directly impact your body's energy levels, metabolism, and overall function. Here's why dietary preparation is vital for biohacking:

- **Energy Production:** The nutrients in the food you consume provide the energy required for all bodily processes, from cellular functions to physical activities.

- **Metabolic Health:** Your diet influences your metabolism, affecting how efficiently your body processes and utilizes nutrients.

- **Nutrient Density:** Biohacking encourages the consumption of nutrient-dense foods that provide essential vitamins, minerals, and antioxidants necessary for optimal health.

Customized Nutrition:

One of the key strengths of biohacking is the customization of nutrition based on individual needs and goals. Dietary preparation involves tailoring your food choices to fit your unique biology and aspirations. This customization includes:

- **Genetic Insights:** Nutrigenomics, the study of how genetics influence nutrition, can inform your dietary choices.

- **Personal Goals:** Whether your aim is weight management, muscle gain, or mental clarity, your diet can be adjusted accordingly.

- **Food Preferences:** Dietary preparation takes into account your personal tastes and preferences, making it more likely that you'll maintain your chosen dietary approach.

Meal Timing and Frequency:

In addition to the types of foods you consume, the timing and frequency of your meals also play a significant role in biohacking. Dietary preparation involves making informed decisions about:

- **Meal Timing:** The timing of your meals can influence energy levels, digestion, and even circadian rhythms. Biohackers often use this information to optimize their daily routines.

- **Intermittent Fasting:** Some biohackers incorporate intermittent fasting, strategically abstaining from food for certain periods, as a way to support metabolic health and longevity.

Addressing Dietary Challenges:

Dietary preparation also involves addressing common dietary challenges that may hinder your biohacking progress. These challenges can include:

- **Food Sensitivities and Allergies:** Identifying and managing food sensitivities or allergies can be a critical part of dietary preparation.

- **Cravings and Emotional Eating:** Strategies for managing cravings and emotional eating are essential for maintaining a healthy diet.

- **Optimizing Digestion:** Ensuring that your body can efficiently digest and absorb nutrients from the foods you eat is crucial for biohacking success.

Sustainable Choices:

Dietary preparation is not just about short-term changes but also about making choices that are sustainable in the long run. A sustainable diet is one that you can maintain over time, supporting ongoing well-being.

- **Behavioral Change:** Preparing your diet for biohacking often involves making gradual behavioral changes that are more likely to stick.

- **Flexible Approaches:** A flexible diet allows for occasional indulgences while still aligning with your health and performance goals.

Dietary preparation is a significant part of laying the groundwork for a successful biohacking journey. By understanding the importance of food as fuel, customization, meal timing, addressing challenges, and sustainability, you can make informed dietary choices that propel you toward better health and a more vibrant life.

The Role of Physical Activity

Physical activity is a crucial aspect of biohacking, impacting not only your physical health but also your mental and emotional well-being. In this section, we'll explore the role of physical activity in biohacking and how it serves as a foundational element for a successful biohacking journey.

Physical Activity and Health:

Physical activity is closely linked to overall health and well-being. Its impact on health is multifaceted and includes the following aspects:

- **Cardiovascular Health:** Regular physical activity improves the health of your heart and circulatory system, reducing the risk of heart disease.

- **Muscular Strength and Endurance:** Engaging in strength training and endurance exercises supports muscle development and resilience.

- **Bone Health:** Weight-bearing activities help maintain bone density and reduce the risk of osteoporosis.

- **Metabolic Function:** Physical activity plays a vital role in metabolic health, influencing how your body processes nutrients and manages blood sugar levels.

Physical Activity and Biohacking:

Biohacking places a strong emphasis on the optimization of physical health and performance. Physical activity is integral to this optimization for several reasons:

- **Performance Enhancement:** Regular exercise can enhance physical performance, whether your goal is to excel in sports, gain strength, or increase endurance.

- **Weight Management:** Physical activity is a powerful tool for weight management, helping to burn calories and build lean muscle.

- **Mood and Mental Clarity:** Exercise has a profound impact on mental and emotional well-being. It can alleviate stress, improve mood, and enhance mental clarity.

- **Longevity and Cellular Health:** Certain forms of exercise, such as high-intensity interval training (HIIT) and resistance training, are associated with longevity and cellular health benefits.

Tailoring Physical Activity:

Biohacking recognizes that physical activity should be tailored to individual needs, goals, and preferences. Here are some key considerations for tailoring your physical activity:

- **Personal Goals:** Whether your focus is on improving cardiovascular health, building strength, or enhancing mental clarity, your choice of physical activity should align with your goals.

- **Body Type and Genetics:** Genetics can influence how your body responds to different forms of exercise. Tailoring your activities based on your genetic profile is a form of personalized biohacking.

- **Lifestyle Integration:** The integration of physical activity into your daily life is essential for long-term sustainability. Biohackers often choose activities that can be seamlessly woven into their routines.

- **Variety:** Combining different types of physical activities, such as aerobic exercise, strength training, and flexibility exercises, can provide a well-rounded approach to fitness.

Data and Progress Tracking:

Biohackers often use data and technology to monitor their physical activity and track progress. Wearable devices, fitness apps, and performance metrics allow for data-driven decision making and the optimization of exercise routines.

- **Quantified Self:** The concept of the "quantified self" involves collecting data on your physical activity, sleep patterns, and other health-related metrics to make informed choices.

- **Setting and Achieving Goals:** Data tracking enables individuals to set specific fitness goals and monitor their progress toward these objectives.

Holistic Well-being:

Physical activity is not isolated from other aspects of well-being. It contributes to a holistic sense of health, encompassing physical, mental, and emotional well-being.

- **Stress Reduction:** Exercise is a potent stress-reduction tool, helping individuals manage the demands of daily life.

- **Energy and Vitality:** Regular physical activity can increase energy levels and promote a sense of vitality.

- **Quality Sleep:** Engaging in physical activity can improve sleep quality, further enhancing overall well-being.

In the realm of biohacking, physical activity is an essential building block for better health, performance, and quality of life. By understanding the multifaceted role of physical activity and tailoring your approach to your individual needs and goals, you can set the stage for a successful biohacking journey.

Prioritizing Quality Sleep

Quality sleep is a cornerstone of successful biohacking, and in this section, we will explore why prioritizing restorative sleep is essential for enhancing your overall well-being.

The Importance of Quality Sleep:

Quality sleep is more than just a period of rest. It is a complex physiological process with profound effects on your health and performance. Prioritizing quality sleep offers various benefits, including:

- **Restoration and Recovery:** During sleep, the body repairs and regenerates tissues, supporting muscle recovery and overall well-being.

- **Cognitive Function:** Adequate sleep is crucial for memory consolidation, problem-solving, and maintaining mental clarity.

- **Mood Regulation:** Sleep plays a significant role in regulating mood and emotional well-being.

- **Immune System Support:** Quality sleep strengthens your immune system, reducing the risk of illness.

Sleep Cycles and Stages:

Understanding the sleep cycle and its stages is vital for optimizing your rest. A typical sleep cycle consists of various stages, including:

- **NREM (Non-Rapid Eye Movement) Stages:** These stages promote physical restoration, growth, and healing.

- **REM (Rapid Eye Movement) Stage:** This stage is associated with vivid dreams and cognitive restoration.

- **Cycle Repetition:** Sleep cycles repeat multiple times during the night.

Factors Affecting Sleep Quality:

Several factors can impact the quality of your sleep. These include:

- **Sleep Environment:** Creating a comfortable sleep environment with a suitable mattress, pillows, and room conditions.

- **Sleep Hygiene:** Practicing good sleep hygiene, including a consistent sleep schedule, can enhance sleep quality.

- **Stress and Anxiety:** Managing stress and anxiety is essential for preventing sleep disturbances.

Biohacking Sleep:

Biohackers explore various techniques to optimize their sleep, such as:

- **Sleep Tracking:** Using wearable devices or apps to monitor sleep patterns and identify areas for improvement.

- **Light and Dark Exposure:** Regulating exposure to light and dark to synchronize your circadian rhythm.

- **Nutrition and Sleep:** Understanding how nutrition can affect sleep quality and adjusting your diet accordingly.

- **Mindfulness and Relaxation Techniques:** Practicing mindfulness and relaxation methods to reduce stress and improve sleep.

Creating a Sleep Routine:

Establishing a consistent sleep routine is a biohacker's strategy for quality sleep:

- **Sleep Schedule:** Set a regular sleep schedule, aiming for the same bedtime and wake-up time every day.

- **Bedtime Rituals:** Develop bedtime rituals that signal your body it's time to sleep.

- **Limiting Stimulants:** Avoiding stimulants, caffeine, and heavy meals close to bedtime.

Prioritizing quality sleep is a fundamental aspect of biohacking, as it contributes to better physical health, cognitive performance, and overall well-being. In the following sections, we will explore techniques to enhance your sleep, monitor your progress, and track your sleep biohacking journey.

Stress Management Techniques

Stress is a common facet of modern life, but biohackers recognize the importance of managing stress effectively. In this section, we will explore stress management techniques and how they contribute to your overall biohacking journey.

Understanding Stress:

Stress can manifest in various forms, including mental, emotional, and physical stress. Recognizing the sources of stress is the first step toward managing it effectively:

- **External Stressors:** These may include work-related pressure, financial concerns, or challenging relationships.

- **Internal Stressors:** Self-imposed expectations and negative thought patterns can contribute to stress.

The Impact of Chronic Stress:

Chronic stress can have detrimental effects on your health and well-being. These include:

- **Physical Health:** Prolonged stress can lead to increased blood pressure, heart disease, and a weakened immune system.

- **Mental Health:** Chronic stress is associated with conditions like anxiety and depression.

- **Cognitive Function:** Stress can impair memory, decision-making, and concentration.

Stress Management Techniques:

Biohackers employ a range of techniques to effectively manage stress:

- **Mindfulness and Meditation:** Mindfulness practices and meditation help you stay present, reduce anxiety, and foster emotional regulation.

- **Breathing Exercises:** Controlled breathing techniques can calm the nervous system and lower stress levels.

- **Exercise:** Regular physical activity releases endorphins, which improve mood and reduce stress.

- **Sleep:** Prioritizing quality sleep is essential for stress management.

- **Nutrition:** A balanced diet supports overall well-being and helps manage stress.

- **Social Connections:** Strong social connections and a support network can help reduce stress.

- **Time Management:** Effective time management and organization can reduce the stress of overwhelming tasks.

- **Biofeedback and Wearable Devices:** Monitoring physiological responses to stress can help you understand your body's reactions and manage stress effectively.

Personalized Stress Management:

Biohackers often personalize their stress management techniques to align with their unique needs and preferences:

- **Stress Triggers:** Identify your individual stress triggers to tailor your stress management approach.

- **Biofeedback Data:** Utilize data from biofeedback devices to fine-tune your stress management strategies.

- **Daily Practices:** Incorporate stress management practices into your daily routine to ensure consistency.

Effectively managing stress is a crucial component of biohacking. By understanding stress, employing a variety of stress management techniques, and personalizing your approach, you can maintain a balanced, stress-free state conducive to optimal health and well-being.

In the upcoming sections, we will delve deeper into other aspects of biohacking, including the role of nutrition and exercise, mental clarity and performance, and the integration of technology in your biohacking journey.

Chapter 5: Building Basic Knowledge: Grasping an Overview of Nutrition and Exercise

The Role of Nutrition in Biohacking

Nutrition is a fundamental pillar of biohacking, as it plays a vital role in optimizing your physical and mental health. In this section, we will explore the central role of nutrition in the biohacking journey.

The Significance of Nutrition:

Nutrition is more than just fuel for the body; it's a complex web of nutrients that impact every facet of your health and well-being. Understanding the significance of nutrition is crucial:

- **Energy Production:** Nutrition provides the energy necessary for daily activities and exercise.

- **Cellular Function:** Nutrients support cellular processes, ensuring optimal function.

- **Hormone Regulation:** Nutrition influences hormone production, affecting mood, energy levels, and overall health.

- **Immune System Support:** Proper nutrition enhances the body's defense against illness and infection.

Nutrients and Biohacking:

Biohackers delve into the world of nutrients, understanding how different components of nutrition impact their health:

- **Macronutrients:** These include carbohydrates, proteins, and fats, each with specific roles in energy, muscle building, and overall health.

- **Micronutrients:** Vitamins and minerals are essential for various bodily functions, from immune support to cognitive function.

- **Phytonutrients and Antioxidants:** These compounds found in plants offer numerous health benefits.

Customized Nutrition:

Biohacking emphasizes personalized nutrition to cater to individual goals and needs:

- **Defining Objectives:** Determine specific goals, whether they're weight management, muscle gain, cognitive enhancement, or overall well-being.

- **Balanced Diets:** Tailor your diet to include a balance of macronutrients, micronutrients, and phytonutrients.

- **Meal Timing:** The timing of meals and nutrient intake can impact energy levels, performance, and metabolism.

- **Nutrition Tracking:** Biohackers often use apps and wearable devices to monitor nutrient intake and its effects on their bodies.

Biohacking Diets:

Biohackers experiment with various diets to find the one that aligns best with their goals. Some popular biohacking diets include:

- **Ketogenic Diet:** Emphasizes high-fat, low-carbohydrate intake, potentially leading to improved fat burning and mental clarity.

- **Intermittent Fasting:** Cycling between eating and fasting periods to support weight loss and metabolic health.

- **Paleolithic Diet (Paleo):** Focuses on whole foods that mimic the diets of our ancestors, excluding processed foods.

The Gut-Brain Connection:

Research shows the strong connection between gut health and mental well-being. Biohackers understand this connection and often seek to improve gut health for optimal cognitive function.

Nutrigenomics:

Nutrigenomics explores how your genetics influence your nutritional needs. Biohackers may use genetic testing to personalize their diets based on their genetic makeup.

Nutrition is a powerful tool in the biohacker's arsenal, shaping both physical health and mental performance. By understanding the significance of nutrition, exploring different nutrients, customizing your diet, and considering biohacking diets, you can optimize your nutrition to support your biohacking goals.

In the upcoming sections, we will delve deeper into the role of exercise in biohacking, the synergy between nutrition and exercise, and practical applications of this knowledge to achieve your biohacking objectives.

The Role of Exercise in Biohacking

Exercise is a cornerstone of biohacking, influencing not only physical health but also mental well-being and cognitive performance. In this section, we will explore the crucial role of exercise in the biohacking journey.

The Significance of Exercise:

Exercise is not just a means to improve physical fitness but a powerful tool to enhance overall well-being. Recognizing the significance of exercise is essential:

- **Physical Health:** Regular exercise supports cardiovascular health, muscle and bone strength, and weight management.

- **Mental Well-Being:** Exercise is linked to reduced stress, anxiety, and depression, fostering mental clarity and emotional regulation.

- **Cognitive Performance:** Physical activity can boost cognitive function, memory, and creativity.

- **Energy Levels:** Regular exercise increases energy levels and overall vitality.

Types of Exercise:

Biohackers explore various forms of exercise to cater to their specific goals and preferences. Some common types of exercise include:

- **Cardiovascular (Aerobic) Exercise:** Activities such as running, swimming, and cycling improve cardiovascular health and endurance.

- **Strength (Resistance) Training:** Resistance exercises, including weightlifting, promote muscle and bone strength.

- **Flexibility and Mobility Training:** Activities like yoga and stretching enhance flexibility and joint mobility.

- **High-Intensity Interval Training (HIIT):** HIIT involves short bursts of intense exercise, known to improve both cardiovascular and metabolic health.

Customized Exercise:

Biohackers personalize their exercise routines to align with their goals and lifestyle:

- **Defining Objectives:** Clearly establish what you aim to achieve with exercise, whether it's weight management, muscle gain, cognitive enhancement, or overall well-being.

- **Exercise Frequency and Duration:** Tailor your exercise routine to fit your schedule and energy levels.

- **Periodization:** Varying the intensity and type of exercise over time can prevent plateaus and enhance progress.

- **Recovery and Rest:** Understanding the importance of rest and recovery in exercise routines is essential for avoiding burnout and injury.

Biohacking Techniques in Exercise:

Biohackers use various techniques to optimize exercise:

- **Tracking and Monitoring:** Wearable devices and apps can monitor exercise performance, providing data for improvement.

- **Biofeedback:** Biofeedback devices measure physiological responses during exercise to inform training strategies.

- **Nutrition and Exercise Synergy:** Coordinating nutrition and exercise can maximize the benefits of both.

Biohacking Workouts:

Biohackers often experiment with specific workout strategies to achieve their goals, such as:

- **Cognitive Enhancing Workouts:** Incorporating cognitive challenges during exercise to enhance mental performance.

- **Recovery Workouts:** Light workouts or practices that focus on recovery and reducing post-exercise soreness.

- **Metabolic Conditioning:** Training that aims to optimize metabolism, improve fat burning, and enhance endurance.

Mental and Physical Synergy:

Exercise not only benefits physical health but also fosters mental clarity, creativity, and overall well-being. Biohackers recognize the synergy between physical and mental performance.

Exercise is a fundamental tool for biohackers, contributing to better physical health, mental well-being, and cognitive performance. By understanding the significance of exercise, personalizing your workout routine, and exploring biohacking techniques, you can leverage exercise to optimize your biohacking journey.

Nutrition and Exercise Synergy

In the world of biohacking, to optimize health, performance, and overall well-

Tailoring Nutrition and Exercise to Your Goals

Biohacking is all about personalization, and this extends to both nutrition and exercise. In this section, we will explore how biohackers tailor their dietary and exercise strategies to align with their unique objectives and goals.

Defining Your Goals:

Biohackers begin by clearly defining their goals. This step is essential to create a customized plan that caters to individual needs. Common biohacking goals include:

- **Weight Management:** Whether it's losing, gaining, or maintaining weight, nutrition and exercise strategies can be tailored accordingly.

- **Muscle Gain:** Those aiming to build muscle will require specific dietary choices and exercise routines.

- **Cognitive Enhancement:** Biohackers looking to boost mental clarity, memory, and cognitive performance will focus on specific nutrients and cognitive-enhancing workouts.

- **Overall Well-Being:** Some individuals prioritize overall health and vitality, with a combination of nutrition and exercise that supports this goal.

Nutrition Strategies:

Once goals are established, biohackers customize their nutrition strategies:

- **Macro Ratios:** Biohackers adjust the proportions of macronutrients (carbohydrates, proteins, and fats) to meet their goals. For instance, a high-protein diet may be chosen for muscle gain.

- **Caloric Intake:** The number of calories consumed can be tailored to match weight management goals.

- **Micronutrient Emphasis:** Biohackers focus on specific vitamins and minerals that support their objectives. For example, omega-3 fatty acids for cognitive enhancement.

- **Meal Timing:** The timing of meals can be adjusted to coordinate with exercise routines and intermittent fasting if desired.

Exercise Strategies:

Exercise routines are also personalized to align with biohacking goals:

- **Type of Exercise:** Cardiovascular, resistance, flexibility, and cognitive-enhancing workouts are chosen based on objectives.

- **Frequency and Duration:** The number of workouts and their duration is determined by the biohacker's schedule and energy levels.

- **Periodization:** Variations in the intensity and type of exercise are introduced to prevent plateaus and enhance progress.

- **Recovery and Rest:** The importance of rest and recovery is recognized to avoid burnout and injury.

Combining Nutrition and Exercise:

Biohackers skillfully combine their nutrition and exercise strategies:

- **Pre-Workout Nutrition:** Meals or snacks are timed to provide energy for productive workouts.

- **Post-Workout Nutrition:** Nutrients support muscle recovery and overall well-being after exercise.

- **Intermittent Fasting:** Some biohackers pair intermittent fasting with exercise to optimize metabolic health and weight management.

Tracking Progress:

Wearable devices, apps, and biofeedback tools play a vital role in tracking and monitoring progress. Data-driven insights help biohackers adjust their strategies for better results.

Adaptation and Flexibility:

Biohackers recognize that goals and circumstances may change. Adaptation and flexibility are crucial for long-term success. Plans are adjusted as needed to stay in line with evolving objectives.

Personalization is the heart of biohacking. By defining clear goals, customizing nutrition and exercise strategies, and staying adaptable, biohackers can effectively harness the power of personalization to achieve their unique objectives.

Practical Application of Nutrition and Exercise Knowledge

Now that we've explored the fundamental principles of nutrition and exercise and how to tailor them to specific goals, it's time to put this knowledge into practice. In this section, we'll provide practical guidance on how to apply your nutrition and exercise strategies effectively for your biohacking journey.

Creating a Nutrition Plan:

A well-crafted nutrition plan is the cornerstone of biohacking success. Here's how to create one:

- **Assess Your Current Diet:** Begin by evaluating your current eating habits. Identify areas that need improvement and understand your nutritional baseline.

- **Set Specific Objectives:** Clearly define your nutritional goals, whether it's weight management, muscle gain, cognitive enhancement, or overall well-being.

- **Balanced Macronutrients:** Ensure your diet includes a balance of carbohydrates, proteins, and fats in proportions that align with your goals.

- **Micronutrient Focus:** Identify specific vitamins and minerals that support your objectives and incorporate foods rich in these nutrients.

- **Meal Timing:** Coordinate your meals with your exercise routine, and consider intermittent fasting if it suits your goals.

- **Dietary Variety:** Include a wide variety of foods to access a broad spectrum of nutrients. Experiment with different sources of proteins, carbohydrates, and fats.

Structuring Your Exercise Routine:

A well-structured exercise routine complements your nutrition plan:

- **Select the Right Exercises:** Choose exercises that match your objectives, whether it's cardiovascular workouts, resistance training, flexibility exercises, or cognitive-enhancing routines.

- **Frequency and Duration:** Determine how often you'll exercise and the duration of each session. Ensure your schedule is sustainable.

- **Progressive Overload:** Gradually increase the intensity or resistance in your workouts to promote continuous improvement.

- **Recovery and Rest:** Prioritize rest days to prevent overtraining and support muscle recovery. Utilize recovery techniques like stretching, foam rolling, and relaxation.

- **Adapt to Your Schedule:** Recognize that life can be unpredictable. Be adaptable and make adjustments when necessary.

Coordination and Timing:

To maximize the synergy between nutrition and exercise:

- **Pre-Workout Nutrition:** Consume a balanced meal or snack before exercise to fuel your workout.

- **Post-Workout Nutrition:** After exercise, provide your body with the nutrients it needs for recovery.

- **Intermittent Fasting:** If you're practicing intermittent fasting, coordinate your eating window with your exercise schedule for metabolic optimization.

Monitoring Progress:

Use technology and biofeedback tools to track your progress. Key steps include:

- **Data Collection:** Record your exercise routines, nutrition, sleep patterns, and other relevant data.

- **Data Analysis:** Regularly review your data to identify trends and areas for improvement.

- **Adjustment:** Based on data-driven insights, make informed adjustments to your nutrition and exercise plans.

Staying Adaptable:

Recognize that biohacking is a dynamic journey. Be open to adaptation and remain flexible in response to changing goals and circumstances.

By practically applying your nutrition and exercise knowledge, you can optimize your well-being and make significant progress in your biohacking journey. The next section will delve into the significance of patience and self-control in the world of biohacking.

Chapter 6: The Importance of Patience and Self-Control

The Nature of Biohacking

To embark on a successful biohacking journey, it's essential to understand the fundamental nature of biohacking. This chapter delves into the core principles, goals, and ethical considerations that define the world of biohacking.

Defining Biohacking:

Biohacking is the practice of self-optimization, driven by a deep desire for enhanced physical, mental, and emotional well-being. At its core, biohacking is about taking control of your biology, making deliberate choices, and utilizing scientific knowledge to achieve your health and performance goals.

The Key Objectives of Biohacking:

Biohackers have a range of goals, including:

- **Improved Health:** Many individuals turn to biohacking as a response to health issues. They seek to address chronic conditions, enhance immune function, or prevent diseases.

- **Enhanced Performance:** Biohackers aim to boost their cognitive performance, physical abilities, and overall energy levels. This may involve optimizing nutrition, exercise, and sleep.

- **Longevity and Quality of Life:** Some are driven by the desire to extend their lifespan and maintain a high quality of life well into old age. Longevity biohacking involves strategies like calorie restriction and lifestyle adjustments.

- **Individual Empowerment:** Biohacking is a path to self-empowerment. It encourages individuals to take charge of their well-being and make informed choices.

- **Personal Goals:** Biohackers may set specific, individualized objectives, such as losing weight, building muscle, or achieving mental clarity.

Ethical Considerations and Safety:

Biohacking is not without ethical concerns. Safety and ethical boundaries are vital aspects of biohacking:

- **Respect for the Body:** Biohackers acknowledge the need to respect the body's natural processes and avoid unnecessary risks.

- **Evidence-Based Practices:** Biohacking is rooted in scientific evidence and responsible experimentation. It does not endorse pseudoscience or unproven methods.

- **Informed Decision-Making:** Informed consent and informed decision-making are crucial. Individuals should thoroughly research and understand the implications of their biohacking choices.

- **Safety Precautions:** Biohackers prioritize safety and monitor their progress to mitigate potential risks.

The Flexibility of Biohacking:

One of the most notable features of biohacking is its adaptability. Biohackers recognize that personal goals and circumstances can evolve. As such, the strategies and techniques they employ are adaptable and adjustable, ensuring continued progress and improvement.

By understanding the nature of biohacking, individuals can make informed choices and embark on a journey that aligns with their objectives and values. In the following sections, we will explore the pitfalls of impatience, the virtue of self-control, and how to develop these critical attributes in the context of biohacking.

The Pitfalls of Impatience

Impatience is a common challenge in the world of biohacking. Many individuals start their journey with high hopes and ambitious goals, only to be derailed by impatience. This section explores the pitfalls of impatience and how it can hinder progress.

The Desire for Quick Results:

Impatience often arises from the desire for quick, noticeable results. In a world of instant gratification, people expect to see significant changes in a short time. Biohacking, however, is a journey that demands patience and persistence.

Overlooking the Importance of Consistency:

Effective biohacking is built on consistent efforts. Small, daily improvements compound over time, leading to significant results. Impatience can lead to a lack of consistency, with individuals giving up too soon if they don't see immediate changes.

Risky Decision-Making:

Impatience can drive individuals to take extreme measures in the pursuit of rapid progress. This can include risky dietary choices, aggressive exercise routines, or the use of untested supplements, all of which can have adverse effects on health.

Unrealistic Expectations:

Impatience often leads to unrealistic expectations. When reality doesn't align with these expectations, it can lead to frustration, disappointment, and a sense of failure.

The Importance of Realistic Timelines:

Biohacking is a long-term journey, and setting realistic timelines is essential. By acknowledging that meaningful change takes time, individuals can better manage their impatience.

Strategies for Overcoming Impatience:

Overcoming impatience is critical for a successful biohacking journey:

- **Set Realistic Goals:** Define achievable, incremental goals that align with your long-term vision.

- **Celebrate Small Wins:** Recognize and celebrate your small successes. This positive reinforcement can help combat impatience.

- **Embrace the Process:** Focus on the journey itself, not just the end result. Find enjoyment and fulfillment in the daily actions you take.

- **Practice Mindfulness:** Mindfulness techniques can help individuals stay present and reduce anxiety about future results.

- **Seek Support:** Joining biohacking communities or working with a coach can provide guidance, accountability, and a sense of camaraderie that helps combat impatience.

The Path to Long-Term Success:

Biohacking is not a sprint; it's a marathon. By recognizing and addressing the pitfalls of impatience, biohackers can stay committed, make steady progress, and achieve sustainable, long-term success.

The next section will delve into the virtue of self-control and how it plays a crucial role in biohacking. If you'd like to continue with the next section or have any specific requests, please feel free to let me know.

The Virtue of Self-Control

Self-control is a cornerstone of successful biohacking. It's the ability to regulate your behavior, thoughts, and emotions to achieve long-term goals and make choices that align with your values. This section explores the vital role of self-control in the biohacking journey.

The Significance of Self-Control:

In the context of biohacking, self-control encompasses several crucial aspects:

- **Dietary Choices:** Self-control helps individuals make healthy food choices and resist the temptation of unhealthy, indulgent options.

- **Exercise Consistency:** It aids in maintaining a regular exercise routine, even when motivation is low.

- **Stress Management:** Self-control allows individuals to employ effective stress management techniques, mitigating the impact of stress on health and performance.

- **Long-Term Vision:** It enables individuals to stay focused on their long-term biohacking goals and make choices that align with those goals.

Resisting Instant Gratification:

Biohacking often involves forgoing instant gratification for long-term gains. This can be challenging in a world where immediate rewards are prevalent. Self-control empowers individuals to resist temptations that may hinder their progress.

Developing Self-Control:

Developing self-control is a skill that can be honed over time. Here are some strategies for enhancing self-control:

- **Set Clear Goals:** Clearly defined goals provide motivation and direction for exercising self-control.

- **Practice Mindfulness:** Mindfulness techniques help individuals become more aware of their impulses and choose healthier responses.

- **Create a Supportive Environment:** Surrounding oneself with a supportive environment that encourages healthy choices can make practicing self-control easier.

- **Reward System:** Establish a reward system that offers positive reinforcement for demonstrating self-control.

- **Learn from Setbacks:** Accept that setbacks will occur, but view them as opportunities for growth and self-improvement.

Biohacking and Self-Control:

Biohacking, by its nature, encourages self-control. It requires making informed choices about nutrition, exercise, and other aspects of well-being. By practicing self-control, biohackers can maintain consistency, avoid impulsive decisions, and stay aligned with their long-term vision.

Balancing Self-Control and Flexibility:

While self-control is essential, it should be balanced with flexibility. Being overly rigid can lead to burnout or frustration. Biohackers should learn when to be disciplined and when to allow themselves some leeway.

The Power of Habit:

Developing healthy habits can make self-control easier. By turning beneficial behaviors into routine habits, individuals can reduce the effort required to exercise self-control.

The next section will explore strategies for developing patience and self-control in the context of biohacking.

Developing Patience and Self-Control

Developing patience and self-control is a continuous process in the world of biohacking. This section delves into strategies and techniques to nurture these virtues and leverage them for long-term success.

Recognizing the Need for Patience and Self-Control:

Before diving into strategies for development, it's essential to understand why patience and self-control are crucial in biohacking:

- **Patience** is required because significant changes in health and well-being take time. It's about embracing the journey and being willing to wait for results.

- **Self-control** is necessary to make informed and healthy choices consistently. It enables biohackers to resist temptations and distractions that may hinder their progress.

Strategies for Developing Patience:

- **Set Realistic Timelines:** Acknowledge that meaningful change takes time. Set realistic expectations and timelines for your biohacking goals.

- **Focus on Small Wins:** Celebrate the small victories along the way. These are indicators of progress and can boost your motivation.

- **Embrace the Learning Process:** Biohacking is about discovering what works for you. Embrace the learning process, even when things don't go as planned.

- **Mindfulness and Meditation:** Practices like mindfulness and meditation can help you stay present and reduce anxiety about future results.

- **Community and Support:** Joining biohacking communities or seeking support from a coach can provide guidance, accountability, and motivation to stay patient.

Strategies for Developing Self-Control:

- **Set Clear Goals:** Clearly define your biohacking goals. Having a clear sense of purpose can help you make choices that align with those goals.

- **Practice Delayed Gratification:** Train yourself to delay instant gratification for long-term rewards. This can be as simple as choosing a healthy snack over a sugary one.

- **Positive Reinforcement:** Reward yourself for demonstrating self-control. Create a reward system that recognizes your efforts.

- **Learn from Setbacks:** Accept that setbacks are a part of any journey. Instead of viewing them as failures, consider them as opportunities for growth.

- **Habit Formation:** Turn beneficial behaviors into routine habits. Habits require less conscious effort, making it easier to exercise self-control.

Finding the Right Balance:

Balancing patience and self-control is essential. Being too rigid can lead to frustration, while being too patient can lead to complacency. Finding the right equilibrium ensures steady progress.

The Path to Sustainable Biohacking:

Both patience and self-control are skills that can be cultivated and strengthened over time. Biohackers who can master these virtues are better equipped to make informed decisions, stay consistent, and achieve sustainable, long-term success in their biohacking journey.

The next section will discuss strategies for navigating plateaus and setbacks in biohacking. If you'd like to continue with the next section or have any specific requests, please feel free to let me know.

Navigating Plateaus and Setbacks

Navigating plateaus and setbacks is an integral part of the biohacking journey. Biohackers often encounter periods where progress stalls or even regresses. This section explores strategies to overcome these challenges and stay on course.

Understanding Plateaus and Setbacks:

- **Plateaus** are phases where biohackers experience a temporary halt in progress despite consistent efforts. They can be frustrating but are a natural part of any improvement process.

- **Setbacks** refer to moments when biohackers face obstacles that hinder their progress. These can range from health issues to lifestyle disruptions.

Strategies for Navigating Plateaus:

- **Evaluate Your Approach:** During plateaus, it's crucial to review your biohacking practices. Consider whether there's a need to change your strategies or try something new.

- **Be Patient:** As mentioned earlier, patience is vital. Plateaus are usually followed by breakthroughs, so stay committed to your goals.

- **Change Your Routine:** Introducing variation to your routine, whether it's in exercise or nutrition, can help overcome plateaus.

- **Set New Goals:** Sometimes, setting new, achievable goals can reignite motivation and break through plateaus.

Strategies for Overcoming Setbacks:

- **Adapt and Modify:** When facing setbacks, be prepared to adapt and modify your biohacking practices to accommodate the changes or challenges you're experiencing.

- **Seek Professional Guidance:** If a setback is due to health issues or specific concerns, consult with a healthcare professional or specialist for guidance.

- **Maintain Resilience:** Setbacks are part of the journey. Maintain resilience and view them as opportunities to learn and grow.

The Role of Support:

Support from biohacking communities, mentors, or friends can be invaluable during plateaus and setbacks. They provide guidance, motivation, and a sense of belonging that can help you stay on track.

Learning and Growth:

Plateaus and setbacks are opportunities for learning and personal growth. They challenge biohackers to refine their approaches, build resilience, and adapt to changing circumstances.

Staying Committed:

Staying committed to your biohacking journey during plateaus and setbacks is a testament to your dedication and resilience. It reinforces the importance of your goals and your determination to achieve them.

Navigating these challenges can be one of the most rewarding aspects of biohacking, as it encourages self-discovery and the development of coping strategies. It also sets the stage for the next chapters in the biohacking journey.

The next section will dive into biohacking through nutrition, focusing on how to choose foods for health and optimal performance.

PART III
Tools and Biohacking Methods

Chapter 7: Biohacking through Nutrition: How to Choose Foods for Health and Optimal Performance

The Power of Nutrition in Biohacking

Nutrition plays a pivotal role in the world of biohacking, shaping health, performance, and longevity. This section delves into the profound impact of nutrition on biohacking and how to harness its power for your well-being.

The Foundation of Health:

Nutrition serves as the cornerstone of health. The foods you consume provide the building blocks for every cell in your body. Understanding this foundation is essential in the world of biohacking.

Fueling Your Body:

- **Macronutrients:** Carbohydrates, proteins, and fats are the primary macronutrients that supply energy and nutrients essential for daily functions.

- **Micronutrients:** Vitamins and minerals act as co-factors for various biochemical processes. They are essential for overall health.

- **Phytonutrients:** These are compounds found in plants that offer additional health benefits. They include antioxidants, anti-inflammatory substances, and more.

The Role of Nutrition in Biohacking:

- **Energy and Focus:** Proper nutrition can enhance energy levels, sharpen mental focus, and stabilize mood.

- **Weight Management:** Nutrition plays a critical role in weight regulation and body composition, making it a vital component of biohacking for those seeking physical improvements.

- **Hormone Balance:** Nutrition can influence hormone balance, impacting everything from stress management to sleep quality.

- **Disease Prevention:** A well-rounded and nutrient-rich diet can reduce the risk of chronic diseases and promote longevity.

Tailoring Nutrition to Biohacking Goals:

Biohackers often have specific goals in mind, whether it's weight loss, muscle gain, enhanced cognition, or longevity. Nutrition can be tailored to align with these objectives. The chapter ahead will explore key principles and strategies for biohacking through nutrition.

A Holistic Approach:

The biohacking approach to nutrition is holistic, considering not just individual nutrients but the synergy between them and the broader impact on the body's systems. This approach allows for a more comprehensive and personalized strategy.

Key Principles of Biohacking Nutrition

Biohacking nutrition revolves around a set of principles that guide the selection of foods to enhance health, performance, and well-being. These principles lay the foundation for a biohacker's dietary strategy.

Nutrient Density:

- **Emphasis on Whole Foods:** Biohackers prioritize whole, unprocessed foods that are rich in essential nutrients. These foods provide more vitamins, minerals, and antioxidants per calorie.

- **Diversity of Nutrients:** A varied diet ensures a broad spectrum of nutrients, supporting the body's multifaceted needs.

Personalization:

- **Bioindividuality:** Recognizing that each person is unique, biohackers tailor their nutrition to their specific needs, goals, and responses to foods.

- **Metabolic Typing:** Some biohackers use metabolic typing to match dietary patterns with their individual metabolic characteristics.

Nutrient Timing:

- **Strategic Eating:** Timing meals to align with circadian rhythms, physical activity, and mental demands can optimize energy and performance.

- **Fasting:** Intermittent fasting and extended fasting periods are explored for potential health benefits, including autophagy and improved insulin sensitivity.

Quality and Sourcing:

- **Organic and Sustainable:** Many biohackers prioritize organic and sustainably sourced foods to minimize exposure to pesticides and support environmental conservation.

- **Food Sensitivities:** Identifying and addressing food sensitivities or allergies to optimize digestion and overall well-being.

Biohacking Supplements:

- **Targeted Supplementation:** Biohackers use supplements strategically to fill nutritional gaps and enhance specific outcomes, such as cognitive function, physical performance, or longevity.

- **Bioavailability:** Selecting supplements with high bioavailability ensures that the body can absorb and utilize them effectively.

Adaptation to Goals:

- **Weight Management:** Nutrition can be adjusted to support weight loss, muscle gain, or body composition changes.

- **Cognitive Enhancement:** Specific nutrients and dietary patterns are explored for enhancing mental clarity, focus, and memory.

Mindful Eating:

- **Sensory Awareness:** Paying close attention to the sensory experience of eating, which can lead to better food choices and satisfaction.

- **Slow Eating:** Eating slowly and savoring each bite can improve digestion and promote satiety.

Tracking and Data Analysis:

- **Self-Monitoring:** Biohackers often use food journals, apps, or wearable devices to track their dietary intake and analyze the impact on their bodies.

- **Feedback Loop:** Analyzing data allows for adjustments and continual refinement of the dietary approach.

These key principles provide a robust framework for biohackers to optimize their nutrition. The next section will delve into the role of micronutrients, which are crucial components of a biohacker's dietary strategy.

The Role of Micronutrients

Micronutrients are the unsung heroes of a biohacker's diet. While they are required in smaller quantities compared to macronutrients, they play a crucial role in various physiological processes and overall well-being.

Understanding Micronutrients:

Micronutrients consist of vitamins and minerals, and they are essential for the proper functioning of the body. They act as co-factors for enzymatic reactions, play a role in energy metabolism, support immune function, and contribute to numerous other processes.

Categories of Micronutrients:

- **Vitamins:** These are organic compounds essential for various bodily functions. For example, vitamin C is critical for collagen production, while vitamin D plays a role in bone health and immune function.

- **Minerals:** These are inorganic elements that are necessary for a range of physiological processes. Examples include calcium for bone health, iron for oxygen transport, and magnesium for muscle function.

Bioavailability:

The body's ability to absorb and utilize micronutrients can vary depending on the source and other factors. Biohackers often seek foods that offer high bioavailability to ensure the body can make the most of these nutrients.

Micronutrients and Biohacking:

- **Cognitive Enhancement:** Specific vitamins and minerals, such as B vitamins and magnesium, are known to support brain function, memory, and focus.

- Immune Support: Micronutrients like vitamin C and zinc are crucial for immune system health and can be employed to reduce the risk of illness or recover faster.

- Anti-Aging: Antioxidant vitamins, such as vitamin E and beta-carotene, are investigated for their potential in slowing down the aging process by neutralizing free radicals.

- Energy Metabolism: B vitamins, particularly B12 and folate, play a significant role in energy production.

Micronutrient-Rich Foods:

Biohackers seek foods rich in micronutrients. For example:

- Leafy Greens: Spinach, kale, and Swiss chard are rich in vitamins K, C, and various minerals.

- Berries: Blueberries and strawberries provide antioxidants and vitamin C.

- Nuts and Seeds: Almonds, sunflower seeds, and walnuts offer healthy fats, vitamins, and minerals.

- Fatty Fish: Salmon and mackerel supply omega-3 fatty acids and vitamin D.

Supplementation:

In some cases, biohackers may turn to supplements to ensure they meet their micronutrient needs. This is especially common for vitamins and minerals that are challenging to obtain through diet alone.

Understanding the role of micronutrients is a crucial part of biohacking through nutrition. The next section will explore how nutrition can be adapted to individual goals, allowing biohackers to fine-tune their dietary strategies.

Adaptation to Individual Goals

Biohacking nutrition isn't one-size-fits-all; it's highly adaptable to meet individual goals, whether that's improving health, enhancing performance, or achieving specific outcomes. Understanding and adapting nutrition to these goals is a fundamental aspect of biohacking.

Weight Management:

- **Weight Loss:** Biohackers who aim to shed excess weight often employ strategies that create a calorie deficit, such as portion control, reduced carbohydrate intake, and regular exercise.

- **Muscle Gain:** Those looking to build muscle may focus on protein-rich foods, resistance training, and adequate calorie intake to support muscle growth.

Cognitive Enhancement:

- **Nootropic Foods:** Biohackers seeking enhanced mental clarity and cognitive function may include nootropic foods in their diet, such as fatty fish for omega-3s and antioxidant-rich berries.

- **Intermittent Fasting:** Some biohackers experiment with intermittent fasting to support brain health and neuroplasticity.

Longevity and Anti-Aging:

- Caloric Restriction: Caloric restriction without malnutrition is a common approach among biohackers aiming for longevity. It may involve nutrient-dense, lower-calorie foods and occasional fasting.

- Anti-Inflammatory Diet: Reducing inflammation through dietary choices can be an essential strategy for anti-aging, including the inclusion of foods like turmeric and green tea.

Energy and Athletic Performance:

- Carbohydrate Cycling: Biohackers interested in optimizing physical performance may adopt carbohydrate cycling to ensure energy availability during workouts.

- Electrolyte Balance: Ensuring proper electrolyte intake can be critical for endurance athletes and those engaged in intense physical activities.

Tailored Dietary Plans:

Biohackers often experiment with various dietary plans to assess their impact on their specific goals. These may include ketogenic diets, paleo diets, Mediterranean diets, and more, depending on individual preferences and responses.

Monitoring and Fine-Tuning:

- Biohackers regularly monitor their dietary intake and analyze data, making adjustments based on the progress they observe.

- Personalized nutrition approaches may involve regular blood tests to assess nutrient levels and hormone profiles.

Adaptation to individual goals ensures that biohackers can maximize the benefits of their dietary choices, whether it's to enhance cognitive function, extend lifespan, improve physical performance, or meet other specific objectives.

The next section will explore the practical application of nutrition and exercise knowledge, providing insights into how biohackers put their nutrition and exercise strategies into action.

The Impact of Meal Timing

Meal timing is a critical aspect of biohacking nutrition. When you eat can have a significant impact on your energy levels, metabolism, and overall well-being.

Circadian Rhythms:

The body's internal clock, known as circadian rhythms, influences various physiological processes. Meal timing aligned with these rhythms can optimize metabolic functions and support overall health.

- **Breakfast:** Many biohackers prioritize a well-balanced breakfast to kickstart metabolism and provide energy for the day.

- **Lunch:** Lunch is typically the largest meal, as the body's metabolism is at its peak during the middle of the day.

- **Dinner:** Having a lighter dinner or finishing your last meal at least a few hours before bedtime can support better sleep and weight management.

Intermittent Fasting:

Intermittent fasting is a biohacking technique that involves cycling between periods of eating and fasting. This approach can promote fat loss, improve insulin sensitivity, and support cellular repair processes.

- 16/8 Method: This involves fasting for 16 hours and eating during an 8-hour window each day.

- 5:2 Method: This approach restricts calorie intake to around 500-600 calories on two non-consecutive days of the week.

Post-Workout Nutrition:

Biohackers engaged in physical performance often focus on optimizing post-workout nutrition. The post-exercise period is a critical time for replenishing glycogen stores and aiding muscle recovery.

- Protein and Carbohydrates: A combination of protein and carbohydrates is commonly recommended to support muscle recovery and replenish energy stores.

- Timing: Consuming this post-workout meal within a specific window after exercise is often emphasized for maximum benefits.

Chrono-Nutrition:

Chrono-nutrition is a biohacking concept that involves aligning meals with circadian rhythms and considering the timing of certain foods to optimize health.

- Chrono-Nutrient Diet: This approach involves consuming specific nutrients at certain times. For example, carbohydrates earlier in the day and fats in the evening.

Biohacking Apps:

Biohackers may use smartphone apps to track meal timing and circadian rhythms to optimize their eating schedule for their specific goals.

Individual Variation:

It's important to note that meal timing may vary based on individual preferences, schedules, and goals. What works for one person may not be optimal for another.

Understanding the impact of meal timing and aligning it with circadian rhythms can be a powerful tool for biohackers looking to optimize their nutrition for health and performance. The next section will delve into emphasizing exercise as a crucial aspect of biohacking. If you'd like to continue with the next section or have any specific requests, please let me know.

Chapter 8: Emphasizing Exercise: Training for Enhanced Health and Physical Fitness

The Significance of Exercise in Biohacking

Exercise is a cornerstone of biohacking, playing a crucial role in enhancing overall health and physical fitness. Biohackers recognize that physical activity is not only vital for a healthy body but also for optimizing various aspects of well-being.

Physical Fitness and Health:

- Regular exercise is associated with improved cardiovascular health, increased lung capacity, and better muscle strength and endurance.

- It helps maintain a healthy weight, reduce the risk of chronic diseases, and promote overall well-being.

Cognitive Enhancement:

Exercise has a profound impact on cognitive function. Biohackers leverage this to enhance mental clarity, focus, and memory.

- *Aerobic Exercise:* Activities like running, swimming, and cycling increase blood flow to the brain, supporting cognitive function.

- *Resistance Training:* Strength training promotes the release of neurotrophic factors, aiding in the growth of brain cells.

Energy and Vitality:

Engaging in regular physical activity boosts energy levels and vitality, a key aspect of biohacking.

- Biohackers often tailor their exercise routines to boost specific aspects of energy, such as cardiovascular endurance, muscular strength, or flexibility.

Hormone Regulation:

Exercise influences hormone levels, including those related to stress, sleep, and appetite. Biohackers use exercise to optimize these hormones for better health and performance.

- *Cortisol Management:* Stress-reducing exercises can help regulate cortisol levels, promoting emotional well-being.

- *Sleep Quality:* Physical activity can improve sleep patterns, leading to better rest and recovery.

Cellular Health:

Exercise supports cellular health and longevity. Biohackers use exercise to activate cellular repair processes.

- *Autophagy:* Exercise can induce autophagy, a process where the body cleans out damaged cells and regenerates new ones.

Personalization:

Biohackers recognize that the ideal exercise regimen can vary greatly among individuals. As such, they personalize their workouts to align with their goals and preferences.

- **High-Intensity Interval Training (HIIT):** Effective for time-efficient workouts and fat loss.

- **Yoga and Meditation:** For stress reduction and mindfulness.

- **Functional Fitness:** To enhance daily activities and reduce the risk of injury.

Quantified Self:

Many biohackers employ wearable devices and smartphone apps to monitor exercise metrics, such as heart rate, sleep patterns, and activity levels.

These devices provide valuable data that biohackers can use to fine-tune their exercise routines for optimal results.

The significance of exercise in biohacking cannot be understated. Whether it's optimizing physical fitness, enhancing cognitive function, regulating hormones, or promoting longevity, exercise is a key tool for biohackers to achieve their health and performance goals.

Key Principles of Biohacking Exercise

Biohackers understand that exercise can be optimized for various goals, whether it's to enhance physical fitness, cognitive function, or overall well-being. To achieve these goals, they adhere to several key principles:

Goal Setting:

- Biohackers begin by setting clear and specific exercise goals. These goals can be related to physical fitness (e.g., building muscle, improving cardiovascular health), cognitive enhancement (e.g., boosting focus and memory), or overall well-being (e.g., reducing stress and promoting mindfulness).

Personalization:

- Exercise routines are personalized to align with individual preferences and needs. Some biohackers prefer high-intensity workouts, while others may opt for low-impact activities like yoga.

Variation:

- Biohackers understand the importance of exercise variety. They include a mix of cardio, strength training, flexibility, and balance exercises in their routines to prevent plateaus and overuse injuries.

Quantification:

- Wearable devices and smartphone apps are used to monitor exercise metrics. Biohackers track heart rate, sleep patterns, calories burned, and other data to quantify the impact of their workouts.

High-Intensity Interval Training (HIIT):

- HIIT is a popular method among biohackers for its time-efficient approach to exercise. It involves short bursts of intense activity followed by brief rest periods.

Strength Training:

- Building muscle through strength training is a common focus for biohackers. They use progressive resistance training to increase muscle mass and strength.

Neuroplasticity Training:

- Biohackers recognize that exercise can promote neuroplasticity, the brain's ability to rewire and adapt. They incorporate exercises that challenge the mind and body, such as balance and coordination drills.

Recovery:

- Adequate recovery is a fundamental principle. Biohackers prioritize rest and sleep to allow the body to repair and grow stronger. Techniques like foam rolling, stretching, and massage may also be used.

Consistency:

- Consistency is key to biohacking exercise. Biohackers establish regular routines and make exercise a non-negotiable part of their daily or weekly schedules.

Tracking Progress:

- Biohackers use data-driven approaches to track progress. They regularly assess fitness metrics, cognitive function, and overall well-being to make informed adjustments to their routines.

Mindfulness and Stress Reduction:

- Exercise is used not only for physical gains but also for reducing stress and promoting mindfulness. Techniques like yoga and meditation are incorporated into exercise routines.

By adhering to these key principles, biohackers can tailor their exercise routines to optimize their health, cognitive function, and physical fitness. The principles of goal setting, personalization, variation, quantification, and recovery are especially crucial in achieving biohacking exercise goals.

Exercise for Cognitive Enhancement

Biohackers recognize that exercise is not only beneficial for physical health but also for optimizing cognitive function. Here, we delve into the ways exercise can be used to enhance mental clarity, focus, and memory:

Neurotrophic Factors:

- Exercise promotes the release of neurotrophic factors, such as brain-derived neurotrophic factor (BDNF). These proteins support the growth and maintenance of brain cells, which is essential for learning and memory.

Increased Blood Flow:

- Aerobic exercises, like running, swimming, and cycling, significantly increase blood flow to the brain. This enhanced blood circulation brings more oxygen and nutrients to brain cells, aiding in cognitive function.

Stress Reduction:

- Engaging in regular physical activity helps reduce stress levels. High-stress states can negatively impact cognitive function, and exercise acts as a natural stress-reliever.

Enhanced Sleep:

- Consistent exercise improves sleep patterns. Quality sleep is crucial for cognitive function, memory consolidation, and overall mental clarity.

Cognitive Challenges:

- Biohackers incorporate exercises that challenge both the body and the mind. Activities like balance training, coordination drills, and activities that require multitasking can stimulate the brain.

Mindfulness and Meditation:

- Biohackers often include mindfulness practices and meditation within their exercise routines. These techniques not only promote mental clarity but also reduce stress and enhance focus.

Consistency:

- Consistency in exercise routines is vital for cognitive enhancement. Biohackers make exercise a regular part of their lives to reap the long-term benefits for cognitive health.

Personalization:

- Recognizing that cognitive enhancement goals can vary, biohackers personalize their exercise routines. Some may prefer activities that emphasize cardiovascular health, while others may focus on balance and coordination for mental agility.

Quantification:

- Many biohackers employ wearable devices and apps to monitor exercise and cognitive metrics. These tools provide valuable data that can be used to fine-tune exercise routines for optimal cognitive benefits.

By embracing these principles, biohackers use exercise not only to enhance physical fitness but also to sharpen their mental acuity. The interplay between exercise and cognitive function is a central aspect of biohacking, enabling individuals to unlock their full cognitive potential.

The next section will explore the personalization of exercise based on individual goals. If you'd like to continue with the next section or have any specific requests, please let me know.

Personalization of Exercise

Biohacking recognizes that exercise is a highly individualized endeavor, and the goals and preferences of individuals can vary widely. To optimize the benefits of exercise, biohackers emphasize personalization:

Goal-Centric Approach:

- The starting point for personalizing exercise is setting clear and specific goals. These goals can be related to physical fitness, cognitive enhancement, weight management, stress reduction, or overall well-being.

Tailored Exercise Routines:

- Biohackers customize their exercise routines to align with their specific goals. For instance, if the goal is to build muscle, strength training exercises are emphasized. In contrast, someone focused on stress reduction might opt for yoga and meditation.

Time and Frequency:

- Personalization extends to the time and frequency of exercise. Some individuals may prefer short, intense workouts, while others may opt for longer, moderate-intensity sessions. The timing of workouts is also adjusted to fit one's daily schedule and energy levels.

Workout Preferences:

- Biohackers take into account personal preferences for exercise. These preferences might include indoor vs. outdoor workouts, group classes vs. solo routines, or high-energy activities vs. mindful practices.

Individual Health Considerations:

- Existing health conditions and considerations are factored into exercise personalization. Biohackers make adaptations to accommodate any limitations or needs, ensuring safety and well-being.

Quantitative Tracking:

- To measure progress and adjust routines, biohackers use data-driven approaches. Wearable devices and apps monitor fitness metrics, such as heart rate, calories burned, and sleep patterns.

Variety and Periodization:

- To prevent plateaus and maintain motivation, exercise routines are periodically varied. Periodization involves changing aspects of workouts, such as intensity, volume, and exercises, to challenge the body and avoid adaptation.

Feedback and Adjustment:

- Personalization is an ongoing process. Biohackers pay attention to their bodies and minds, seeking feedback on the effectiveness of their routines. When necessary, they make adjustments to optimize results.

Long-Term Sustainability:

- Personalized exercise routines are designed with long-term sustainability in mind. Biohackers aim for routines that can be maintained throughout their lives, promoting continued health and well-being.

By personalizing exercise routines, biohackers ensure that their efforts are aligned with their unique goals and preferences. This individualized approach enhances motivation and makes exercise a sustainable and enjoyable aspect of their biohacking journey.

The Importance of Recovery

In the realm of biohacking exercise, recovery plays a crucial role. Biohackers understand that recovery is not merely downtime but a fundamental aspect of optimizing physical and mental well-being:

Muscle Repair and Growth:

- Recovery is essential for muscle repair and growth. During exercise, muscle tissues experience micro-tears. Adequate recovery time allows these tears to heal and promotes muscle growth, strength, and endurance.

Hormonal Balance:

- Exercise stimulates the release of various hormones, including cortisol and adrenaline. These hormones are crucial for workouts but need to return to baseline levels for overall health. Recovery helps in maintaining hormonal balance.

Injury Prevention:

- Overtraining can lead to injuries. Biohackers recognize the importance of recovery in injury prevention. Rest periods between intense workouts reduce the risk of overuse injuries and strains.

Mental Refreshment:

- Recovery is not only about physical rest but also mental refreshment. It helps reduce exercise-induced stress, improve mood, and maintain cognitive function.

Sleep Quality:

- Adequate recovery, especially through proper sleep, significantly impacts exercise benefits. Sleep is when the body repairs and regenerates, making it a vital aspect of recovery.

Nutrition and Hydration:

- Recovery includes attention to post-workout nutrition and hydration. Consuming the right nutrients and staying hydrated aids in muscle repair and overall recovery.

Adaptation and Progress:

- Biohackers understand that the body adapts and becomes stronger during recovery. The adaptation phase is essential for long-term progress and achieving biohacking goals.

Active Recovery:

- Active recovery techniques, such as light exercise, stretching, and yoga, are used by biohackers to support muscle recovery and reduce soreness.

Individualization:

- Recovery strategies are individualized based on factors like age, fitness level, and specific goals. Personalized recovery plans ensure optimal results.

Quantification:

- Just as with exercise, biohackers use quantification tools to monitor recovery metrics. These tools can include sleep trackers, heart rate variability measurements, and stress level assessments.

Incorporating effective recovery strategies into their exercise routines allows biohackers to maximize the benefits of their efforts while minimizing the risk of burnout, injury, and mental fatigue. The synergy between exercise and recovery is a central tenet of biohacking for enhanced health and physical fitness.

Chapter 9: Focusing on the Mind: How to Boost Mental Clarity and Mental Performance

The Significance of Mental Clarity and Performance

Biohackers recognize that mental clarity and performance are integral components of overall well-being. The mind is a powerful tool, and optimizing its function can have a profound impact on daily life and biohacking goals:

Cognitive Function:

- Mental clarity is closely tied to cognitive function. Biohackers aim to enhance memory, attention, problem-solving abilities, and creativity through various strategies.

Productivity and Efficiency:

- A clear and focused mind leads to increased productivity and efficiency. Biohackers understand that improved mental performance can lead to more effective work and a greater sense of accomplishment.

Stress Reduction:

- Enhanced mental clarity can help reduce stress and anxiety. Biohackers employ techniques that calm the mind and promote relaxation to counteract the effects of a fast-paced, modern lifestyle.

Decision-Making and Problem Solving:

- Mental clarity is vital for making sound decisions and solving complex problems. Biohackers work on strategies to improve decision-making and analytical skills.

Emotional Resilience:

- Mental clarity contributes to emotional resilience. Biohackers seek ways to manage and regulate emotions effectively, fostering a positive outlook and emotional stability.

Optimal Sleep:

- Quality sleep is foundational to mental clarity. Biohackers prioritize sleep hygiene and aim to improve sleep patterns to maximize cognitive function.

Nutrition and Brain Health:

- Nutrition plays a crucial role in mental clarity. Biohackers understand that a balanced diet rich in brain-boosting nutrients supports optimal brain function.

Mind-Body Connection:

- Biohackers explore the profound connection between mental and physical well-being. Techniques such as mindfulness, meditation, and biofeedback are used to enhance this connection.

Personalization:

- Strategies for boosting mental clarity and performance are personalized to individual goals and challenges. Biohackers tailor their approaches to address specific areas of improvement.

Long-Term Brain Health:

- Biohackers view mental clarity as an integral aspect of long-term brain health. Strategies are designed to support cognitive function well into the future.

Enhancing mental clarity and performance is not a one-size-fits-all endeavor. Biohackers employ a variety of techniques and technologies to optimize their mental faculties, ultimately contributing to a higher quality of life and improved problem-solving capabilities.

Key Principles of Biohacking Mental Clarity

Biohackers employ specific principles and techniques to enhance mental clarity and cognitive performance. These principles serve as a foundation for optimizing the mind:

Neuroplasticity:

- Biohackers understand the concept of neuroplasticity, which refers to the brain's ability to reorganize and adapt. They engage in activities that promote neuroplasticity, such as learning new skills and engaging in challenging mental tasks.

Brain-Boosting Nutrition:

- Nutrition plays a vital role in mental clarity. Biohackers focus on consuming foods rich in nutrients that support brain health, including omega-3 fatty acids, antioxidants, and essential vitamins.

Hydration and Cognitive Function:

- Staying adequately hydrated is essential for cognitive function. Biohackers recognize the importance of hydration in maintaining mental clarity and vigilance.

Sleep Optimization:

- Quality sleep is a cornerstone of mental clarity. Biohackers prioritize sleep hygiene, create optimal sleep environments, and adhere to sleep schedules to maximize cognitive function.

Stress Management:

- Stress negatively impacts mental clarity. Biohackers practice stress management techniques, such as meditation and deep breathing exercises, to reduce stress and enhance mental performance.

Mindfulness and Meditation:

- Biohackers often incorporate mindfulness and meditation practices into their daily routines. These practices promote a clear and focused mind and improve emotional well-being.

Cognitive Enhancement Exercises:

- Engaging in cognitive enhancement exercises, such as puzzles, brain training apps, and memory games, is a common strategy among biohackers to sharpen mental acuity.

Biofeedback and Self-Monitoring:

- Biohackers use biofeedback devices and self-monitoring tools to track various metrics related to mental performance, including heart rate variability, brainwave patterns, and stress levels.

Nootropics and Smart Supplements:

- Some biohackers explore the use of nootropics and smart supplements, which are substances believed to enhance cognitive function. They do so with careful consideration and research.

Mind-Body Connection:

- The connection between mental and physical health is acknowledged by biohackers. They integrate physical exercise and relaxation techniques to support overall well-being.

Personalization:

- Biohackers understand that mental clarity needs a personalized approach. They tailor their strategies to address specific areas of improvement and adapt techniques to suit individual goals.

Biohackers are dedicated to continuously improving mental clarity and cognitive performance through a combination of these principles. By focusing on these core elements, they aim to achieve heightened mental acuity, increased productivity, and a greater sense of well-being.

Sleep and Mental Clarity

The connection between sleep and mental clarity is profound, and biohackers recognize the critical role of quality sleep in achieving and maintaining optimal cognitive function. Here, we explore this relationship in more detail:

Sleep Stages and Cognitive Function:

- Biohackers understand that sleep consists of various stages, including deep sleep (slow-wave sleep) and REM (rapid eye movement) sleep. These stages play a crucial role in memory consolidation, learning, and problem-solving. By optimizing their sleep cycles, biohackers aim to improve cognitive function.

Sleep Quantity and Quality:

- Both the quantity and quality of sleep matter. Biohackers prioritize getting the recommended 7-9 hours of sleep each night and create a sleep-conducive environment to enhance sleep quality.

Sleep Hygiene:

- Sleep hygiene practices, such as maintaining a regular sleep schedule, avoiding stimulants before bedtime, and keeping the bedroom cool and dark, are key components of biohackers' routines to ensure restorative sleep.

Sleep Tracking and Monitoring:

- Biohackers use sleep tracking devices and apps to monitor their sleep patterns. By analyzing this data, they can identify areas for improvement and adjust their sleep strategies accordingly.

Sleep as a Cognitive Reset:

- Sleep serves as a cognitive reset button. During deep sleep, the brain undergoes processes that remove waste products and enhance overall cognitive function. Biohackers appreciate the importance of this nightly reset.

Sleep and Emotional Well-Being:

- Sleep has a direct impact on emotional well-being. Biohackers recognize that insufficient sleep can lead to increased stress, irritability, and reduced emotional resilience. Restorative sleep contributes to a positive outlook.

Circadian Rhythms:

- Circadian rhythms, the body's internal clock, influence sleep-wake cycles. Biohackers align their daily routines with these rhythms to improve sleep quality and promote mental clarity.

Napping Strategies:

- Some biohackers explore strategic napping as a way to enhance alertness and mental clarity during the day. They tailor their naps to avoid grogginess and maximize productivity.

Nutrition and Sleep:

- Nutrition plays a role in sleep quality. Biohackers choose foods and nutrients that support better sleep patterns, such as those rich in tryptophan, magnesium, and melatonin precursors.

Cognitive Function After Sleep:

- Biohackers are aware of the phenomenon of sleep inertia, which is the grogginess that can follow awakening. They employ techniques to minimize sleep inertia's impact on cognitive function.

By optimizing their sleep, biohackers aim to enhance mental clarity, improve memory, boost problem-solving abilities, and reduce stress. The next section will explore the mind-body connection and its influence on mental performance.

Mind-Body Connection

The mind-body connection is a central focus in the world of biohacking, recognizing that the state of your body can significantly impact your mental performance. In this section, we explore the various aspects of this connection:

Physical Activity and Cognitive Function:

- Biohackers understand that regular physical activity can enhance cognitive function. They engage in activities such as aerobic exercise and strength training to improve blood flow to the brain and stimulate the release of neurotransmitters associated with mood and cognitive performance.

Nutrition and Brain Health:

- The foods you consume have a direct impact on brain health. Biohackers choose a diet rich in brain-boosting nutrients such as omega-3 fatty acids, antioxidants, and phytochemicals to support mental clarity and focus.

Gut-Brain Axis:

- The gut-brain axis is a bidirectional communication system between the gut and the brain. Biohackers recognize the importance of gut health in mental performance and experiment with probiotics and dietary choices to optimize this connection.

Stress Management and Mental Resilience:

- Chronic stress can negatively affect cognitive function. Biohackers employ stress management techniques like mindfulness, meditation, and deep breathing exercises to reduce the impact of stress on the brain.

Sleep and Emotional Regulation:

- A well-rested body is better equipped to manage emotions and stress. Biohackers prioritize quality sleep to enhance emotional regulation and mental clarity.

Biofeedback and Mindfulness:

- Biohackers explore biofeedback devices and mindfulness practices to gain insights into their physiological responses to stress and emotions. This awareness helps them make real-time adjustments for better mental performance.

Mental Training and Brain Games:

- Cognitive training exercises and brain games are tools that biohackers use to sharpen mental acuity, memory, and problem-solving skills.

Neurofeedback and Brainwave Optimization:

- Some biohackers experiment with neurofeedback and brainwave optimization technologies to modulate brain activity and enhance cognitive function.

Hydration and Cognitive Performance:

- Dehydration can lead to cognitive impairment. Biohackers maintain proper hydration to support optimal brain function.

Mindfulness and Presence:

- Mindfulness practices, such as meditation and yoga, are part of the biohacker's toolkit to increase awareness, reduce mental clutter, and enhance mental performance.

By focusing on the mind-body connection, biohackers aim to achieve mental clarity, emotional balance, and overall cognitive optimization. The next section will delve into personalized approaches to mental performance.

Personalized Approaches

Biohacking acknowledges that one size does not fit all when it comes to enhancing mental clarity and performance. In this section, we delve into the personalized approaches that biohackers utilize to optimize their mental faculties:

Bioindividuality:

- Biohackers recognize that each individual is unique, and what works for one person may not work for another. They embrace the concept of bioindividuality, tailoring their biohacking strategies to their specific genetic makeup, lifestyle, and health conditions.

Personalized Nutrition:

- Biohackers may undergo genetic testing to identify nutritional deficiencies and genetic predispositions. This information helps them create personalized diets that cater to their specific needs, ensuring optimal brain function.

Mindfulness and Cognitive Behavioral Therapy:

- Personalized approaches to mental performance may involve mindfulness techniques and cognitive behavioral therapy tailored to an individual's specific cognitive and emotional challenges.

Neurofeedback Protocols:

- Biohackers who use neurofeedback often customize protocols to address their unique brainwave patterns and target areas for improvement.

Tracking and Self-Monitoring:

- Personalization often involves meticulous tracking of mental performance through the use of journals, apps, and wearable devices. Biohackers collect data on their cognitive abilities and use this information to make informed adjustments.

Goal-Oriented Strategies:

- Personalized approaches align with an individual's specific goals, whether it's improving memory, creativity, problem-solving, or focus. Biohackers craft strategies designed to achieve these objectives.

Cognitive Stack Design:

- Some biohackers develop cognitive stacks, a combination of supplements, nootropics, and lifestyle practices tailored to their cognitive goals.

Feedback Loops:

- Feedback loops involve a constant cycle of monitoring, analyzing data, making changes, and reassessing. Biohackers employ feedback loops to continually fine-tune their mental performance strategies.

Holistic Wellness Integration:

- Biohackers often integrate mental performance strategies into their overall wellness plans. A holistic approach ensures that mental optimization aligns with physical health and emotional well-being.

Biohacking Communities:

- Some biohackers seek out like-minded communities and expert guidance to fine-tune their personalized approaches to mental clarity and performance.

By embracing personalized approaches, biohackers aim to optimize their mental performance in a way that is uniquely suited to their individual needs and aspirations. The next section will explore the utilization of technology in biohacking.

Chapter 10: Utilizing Technology in Biohacking: Useful Smartphone Apps and Tools

The Role of Technology in Biohacking

In the modern era, technology plays a pivotal role in the practice of biohacking. It serves as a powerful enabler, providing biohackers with a plethora of tools, data, and resources to enhance their overall well-being. This section explores the fundamental role of technology in biohacking:

Data Collection and Analysis:

- Technology enables biohackers to collect and analyze a vast amount of data related to their health, performance, and lifestyle. This includes wearable devices that track heart rate, sleep patterns, activity levels, and more. Smartphone apps and specialized tools assist in recording and making sense of this data.

Personalization and Precision:

- Advanced algorithms and machine learning models empower biohackers to personalize their strategies. These technologies can process data to provide insights into what works best for an individual's unique biology and goals.

Biofeedback Devices:

- Biofeedback tools, often connected to smartphones, offer real-time data on various bodily functions. These include heart rate variability, stress levels, and brainwave patterns. Biohackers use this data to make instant adjustments in their routines.

Virtual Health Communities:

- Online platforms, forums, and social networks have given rise to virtual health communities. Biohackers can connect with like-minded individuals, share experiences, and seek guidance from experts worldwide.

Access to Information:

- Smartphones provide instant access to a wealth of information on nutrition, exercise, and health strategies. Biohackers can stay updated with the latest research and trends, helping them make informed choices.

Biohacking Apps:

- Smartphone apps designed for biohacking are prevalent. These apps offer features such as tracking nutrition, exercise, sleep, and mental performance. They also provide biofeedback, goal setting, and reminders to maintain consistency.

Wearable Devices:

- Wearable technology, like fitness trackers and smartwatches, monitors vital signs and activities, making it easier for biohackers to maintain an awareness of their physical and mental states throughout the day.

Biohacking Gadgets:

- Specialized biohacking devices, often smartphone-compatible, offer various functionalities, from light therapy to neurostimulation, designed to enhance mental and physical performance.

Gamification:

- Gamification strategies, implemented through apps and devices, can turn biohacking into an engaging and motivating experience. Achievements, challenges, and rewards help individuals stay committed to their biohacking goals.

Biosecurity and Privacy:

- As technology advances, biohackers also need to be mindful of biosecurity and privacy concerns. Protecting personal data and ensuring the safety of biohacking practices are essential considerations.

Incorporating technology into biohacking opens up a world of possibilities for self-improvement and optimal health. The next section will focus on choosing the right smartphone apps for biohacking. If you'd like to continue with the next section or have any specific requests, please let me know.

Choosing the Right Smartphone Apps

Selecting the appropriate smartphone apps is a critical step in your biohacking journey. These apps can aid in data tracking, performance optimization, and maintaining your overall well-being. In this section, we will explore the factors to consider when choosing the right smartphone apps for biohacking:

Goal Alignment:

- Identify your specific biohacking goals. Are you aiming to improve sleep quality, enhance mental clarity, optimize nutrition, or track physical performance? Choose apps that align with your objectives to ensure they provide relevant data and guidance.

User-Friendly Interface:

- Look for apps with intuitive and user-friendly interfaces. The easier it is to navigate and use the app, the more likely you'll stay consistent in recording your biohacking data.

Compatibility:

- Ensure that the app is compatible with your smartphone's operating system (iOS or Android) and version. This compatibility ensures a smooth experience.

Data Accuracy:

- Verify the accuracy of the data collected by the app. Read user reviews, consult experts, and assess the app's reputation for providing precise measurements and feedback.

Data Security and Privacy:

- Review the app's privacy policy and data security measures. Ensure that your personal and health information is protected and that the app complies with data protection regulations.

Customization:

- Seek apps that allow for customization. The ability to tailor the app to your specific goals and preferences is valuable in biohacking.

Compatibility with Wearable Devices:

- If you use wearable technology, check if the app is compatible with your devices. Integration with your fitness tracker or smartwatch can streamline data collection.

Community and Support:

- Some apps offer community features where you can connect with other biohackers, share experiences, and seek advice. Consider whether you value this aspect in your app choice.

Updates and Support:

- Opt for apps that receive regular updates and have responsive customer support. This ensures that the app remains reliable and functional over time.

Cost:

- Evaluate the cost of the app, including any subscription fees. Some biohacking apps offer both free and premium versions with additional features. Assess whether the features justify the price.

Integration:

- Consider how the app integrates with other apps and services. Integration can simplify the tracking and analysis of your biohacking data.

User Reviews and Recommendations:

- Read user reviews and seek recommendations from the biohacking community. Real-world experiences can offer valuable insights into the effectiveness and usability of different apps.

Choosing the right smartphone apps for biohacking is a personalized process, dependent on your specific goals and preferences. The next section will cover sleep tracking apps, a crucial tool in monitoring sleep quality and patterns.

Sleep Tracking Apps

Quality sleep is a cornerstone of biohacking for optimal health and performance. Monitoring your sleep patterns can provide valuable insights into the duration, quality, and consistency of your rest. Sleep tracking apps are an essential tool in this aspect of biohacking. In this section, we will explore the features to consider when selecting a sleep tracking app:

Comprehensive Sleep Metrics:

- Choose a sleep tracking app that provides comprehensive sleep metrics. This includes data on total sleep time, sleep stages (such as REM and deep sleep), wake times, and disturbances.

Ease of Use:

- Look for apps with an intuitive and easy-to-use interface. The app should make it effortless to start and stop sleep tracking, and to access your sleep data.

Data Visualization:

- Visual representations of your sleep data, such as graphs and charts, can help you quickly understand your sleep patterns. A well-visualized app can aid in identifying trends and areas for improvement.

Smart Alarms:

- Some sleep tracking apps feature smart alarms that wake you up during your lightest sleep phase, which can lead to a more refreshed feeling upon waking.

Compatibility with Wearable Devices:

- If you use a wearable sleep tracker or a smartwatch, choose an app that syncs with your device to provide even more detailed sleep insights.

Sleep Improvement Suggestions:

- Certain apps offer personalized recommendations for improving your sleep based on your data. These can include tips on optimizing your sleep environment and bedtime routines.

Integration with Health and Wellness Apps:

- Consider how the sleep tracking app integrates with other health and wellness apps you use. Integration can provide a more holistic view of your overall well-being.

Data Security:

- Ensure that the app's data handling practices are secure and that your sleep data remains private and confidential.

Reviews and Ratings:

- Reading user reviews and checking app ratings can offer valuable insights into the real-world performance of the sleep tracking app.

Cost:

- Some sleep tracking apps are free, while others offer premium features at a cost. Assess whether the premium features are necessary for your goals.

Updates and Support:

- Opt for apps that are regularly updated and supported by the developer, ensuring the app remains reliable over time.

Sleep tracking apps are invaluable for assessing and improving your sleep patterns, contributing to enhanced overall well-being. The next section will focus on nutrition and diet apps, helping you make informed choices about what you eat.

Nutrition and Diet Apps

Diet and nutrition play a fundamental role in biohacking. What you eat has a direct impact on your health, performance, and well-being. Nutrition and diet apps are invaluable tools for tracking and optimizing your dietary choices. In this section, we will explore the features to consider when selecting a nutrition and diet app:

Food Database:

- Look for apps with a comprehensive food database that allows you to easily search for and log the foods you consume. The database should include a wide range of foods and their nutritional content.

Nutrient Tracking:

- A good nutrition app should allow you to track macronutrients (carbohydrates, proteins, and fats) and micronutrients (vitamins and minerals) to ensure you're meeting your dietary goals.

Meal Planning and Logging:

- Choose an app that lets you plan your meals and log what you eat. Some apps offer meal planning features that help you create balanced and goal-specific meal plans.

Barcode Scanner:

- Apps with barcode scanning capabilities make it easy to log packaged foods accurately. Scan the barcode, and the app will populate the nutritional information for you.

Customized Goals:

- Personalization is key in biohacking. Look for apps that allow you to set and track customized dietary goals, whether you're aiming for weight loss, muscle gain, or improved health.

Meal Analysis:

- Some apps offer meal analysis, which breaks down the nutritional content of your meals and provides insights into their overall healthfulness.

Allergen and Dietary Restriction Support:

- If you have food allergies or dietary restrictions, ensure the app can accommodate these needs by tracking allergens and specific dietary requirements.

Water and Hydration Tracking:

- Proper hydration is often overlooked. Choose an app that includes water and hydration tracking to help you maintain optimal fluid intake.

Integration with Fitness Apps:

- If you use fitness or activity tracking apps, consider how well the nutrition app integrates with them to provide a holistic view of your health.

Community and Support:

- Some nutrition apps have community features or offer access to dietitians and nutritionists for additional support.

Cost:

- Evaluate whether the app is free or offers premium features at a cost. Consider if the premium features align with your specific biohacking and dietary goals.

Data Security:

- Ensure that the app's data handling practices are secure and that your dietary information remains private and confidential.

Choosing the right nutrition and diet app is a critical step in your biohacking journey. The next section will focus on meditation and mindfulness apps, which can enhance your mental well-being.

Meditation and Mindfulness Apps

Meditation and mindfulness are essential components of a comprehensive biohacking toolkit. These practices can help you manage stress, improve focus, and enhance overall well-being. Meditation and mindfulness apps offer structured guidance and support to incorporate these practices into your daily routine. In this section, we will explore key considerations when selecting a meditation and mindfulness app:

Guided Meditation:

- Look for apps that offer a variety of guided meditation sessions, each targeting different aspects of mental well-being, such as stress reduction, focus improvement, or sleep enhancement.

Meditation Timer:

- An essential feature is a meditation timer that allows you to set a specific duration for your meditation sessions, whether it's a brief five minutes or a more extended practice.

Mindfulness Tools:

- The app should provide tools for practicing mindfulness throughout the day, such as breathing exercises and mindfulness reminders.

Progress Tracking:

- The ability to track your meditation progress, set goals, and visualize improvements can be motivating and help you stay consistent.

Sleep and Relaxation Aids:

- Some meditation apps include sleep stories, relaxation exercises, and soothing sounds to help you unwind and improve sleep quality.

Customization:

- Personalization is crucial. Choose an app that lets you tailor your meditation experience to your preferences, whether it's through the selection of instructors, meditation types, or background sounds.

Community and Support:

- Some apps offer a community aspect where you can connect with others, share experiences, and receive guidance from meditation experts.

Offline Access:

- Consider whether the app allows you to download meditation sessions for offline use, which can be especially useful when you're in areas with limited internet connectivity.

Cost:

- Evaluate whether the app is free or offers premium features at a cost. Determine if the premium features align with your specific meditation and mindfulness goals.

Data Security:

- Ensure that the app's data handling practices are secure and that your meditation and mindfulness information remains private and confidential.

Meditation and mindfulness apps can be powerful tools for improving your mental clarity and emotional well-being. The next section will focus on biofeedback and wearable devices, which can provide real-time data to support your biohacking efforts.

Biofeedback and Wearable Devices

Biofeedback and wearable devices have revolutionized the way we monitor and optimize our health and performance. These devices provide real-time data on various physiological parameters, allowing us to gain insights into our body's responses to different stimuli and interventions. In this section, we will explore the key aspects to consider when incorporating biofeedback and wearable devices into your biohacking journey:

Types of Biofeedback and Wearable Devices:

- Understand the different types of devices available, such as heart rate monitors, electroencephalography (EEG) headsets, skin temperature sensors, and more. Select the device that aligns with your specific biohacking goals.

Data Accuracy:

- Ensure that the device you choose provides accurate and reliable data. Read reviews, consult experts, and check for any certifications or validations of the device's accuracy.

Compatibility:

- Verify that the device is compatible with your smartphone and other devices you use for biohacking. It should seamlessly integrate with your existing technology ecosystem.

Real-Time Feedback:

- One of the primary advantages of biofeedback and wearables is real-time data. Look for devices that offer immediate feedback and data visualization.

User-Friendly Interface:

- The accompanying app or software should be user-friendly, making it easy to interpret the data and track your progress.

Customization:

- Some devices allow you to customize the data parameters you want to monitor. Choose devices that align with your biohacking objectives.

Long-Term Use:

- Consider the durability and battery life of the device, especially if you plan to use it for an extended period. A longer battery life can minimize interruptions in data collection.

Data Security:

- Ensure that the device's data transmission and storage practices are secure and compliant with privacy standards.

Cost:

- Evaluate the cost of the device and any associated subscription fees for premium features or services. Make sure it fits within your budget.

Expert Guidance:

- Seek guidance from biohacking experts or healthcare professionals to understand how to interpret the data and make informed decisions based on the information collected.

Biofeedback and wearable devices are valuable tools for biohackers, providing actionable insights and supporting data-driven decision-making. The next section will delve into creating a personal biohacking plan to structure your biohacking journey.

Personalization and Integration

Personalization and integration play a pivotal role in successful biohacking. The ability to tailor your biohacking approach to your individual needs and goals, and seamlessly integrate various tools and techniques, is essential for maximizing the benefits of biohacking. In this section, we will explore the concepts of personalization and integration:

Personalization:

- Recognize that biohacking is not a one-size-fits-all endeavor. It should be personalized to your unique goals, preferences, and requirements. Understanding your individual physiology and genetics can guide you in making targeted choices.

Goal Setting:

- Define clear and specific biohacking goals. Whether you aim to optimize physical performance, enhance cognitive function, improve sleep, or achieve a specific health outcome, your goals will drive your biohacking strategy.

Data-Driven Decision-Making:

- Utilize the data collected from biofeedback and wearable devices, nutrition and exercise tracking, and other tools to inform your decisions. Data-driven biohacking allows you to assess the effectiveness of your interventions.

Iterative Approach:

- Understand that biohacking is an ongoing journey. Continuously assess your progress, adapt your strategies, and refine your biohacking techniques as you learn more about what works best for you.

Holistic Approach:

- Consider the holistic impact of your biohacking efforts. How do nutrition, exercise, sleep, and stress management work together to optimize your well-being? Integration is the key to achieving synergy among these factors.

Lifestyle Integration:

- Incorporate biohacking practices seamlessly into your daily life. The most effective biohacking is not disruptive; it enhances your life without becoming a burden.

Expert Guidance:

- Seek advice from biohacking experts, medical professionals, and nutritionists to ensure that your biohacking approach aligns with your health and safety. They can also provide insights into personalized strategies.

Self-Experimentation:

- Be open to self-experimentation and discovery. You may need to try various approaches to determine what works best for you. Keep detailed records of your experiments and outcomes.

Mindset and Consistency:

- Maintain a positive and growth-oriented mindset. Consistency is crucial in biohacking. It's a long-term commitment to achieving your best self.

Ethical Considerations:

- Consider the ethical implications of your biohacking practices. Respect your own boundaries and the well-being of others as you pursue your biohacking journey.

Personalization and integration are the cornerstones of effective biohacking. They enable you to optimize your health, performance, and well-being in a way that aligns with your unique needs and objectives. The following section will guide you in creating a personal biohacking plan, helping you put these principles into action.

PART IV
Practicing Biohacking and Tracking Progress

Chapter 11: Creating a Personal Biohacking Plan

The Importance of a Personal Biohacking Plan

A personal biohacking plan is the roadmap to your journey of self-improvement and optimization. It's a structured approach that outlines your biohacking goals, strategies, and how you intend to achieve them. In this section, we delve into the significance of creating a personalized biohacking plan:

Goal Clarity:

- Your personal biohacking plan serves as a beacon, illuminating your specific goals. It forces you to clarify what you want to achieve through biohacking, whether it's improved physical performance, mental clarity, longevity, or a combination of these.

Strategy Selection:

- The plan guides you in selecting the biohacking strategies that align with your goals. By understanding the array of options available, you can make informed choices about what to include in your biohacking toolkit.

Individual Tailoring:

- Your biohacking plan is uniquely yours. It tailors your approach to your individual needs, taking into account factors such as your genetics, current health status, lifestyle, and personal preferences.

Prioritization:

- It helps you prioritize your biohacking efforts. Not all biohacking strategies will be equally relevant to your goals. Your plan ensures that you focus your energy and resources on what matters most to you.

Long-Term Perspective:

- A personal biohacking plan encourages you to take a long-term perspective. Biohacking is not a quick fix; it's a journey of continuous improvement. Your plan reminds you of the need for consistency and persistence.

Accountability:

- By documenting your plan, you create a sense of accountability to yourself. This can be a powerful motivator to stick to your biohacking practices and track your progress.

Adaptation:

- Your biohacking plan isn't static. It evolves with you. As you learn more about what works best for you, you can adjust your plan to stay aligned with your goals and changing circumstances.

Data Collection and Analysis:

- It outlines how you will collect and analyze data related to your biohacking interventions. This data-driven approach helps you understand what is working and what isn't.

Tracking Progress:

- Your personal biohacking plan includes mechanisms for monitoring your progress. Tracking your results enables you to stay on course and make data-informed adjustments.

Ethical Considerations:

- Consider the ethical implications of your biohacking plan, ensuring that your practices respect your well-being and the well-being of others.

Your personal biohacking plan is a dynamic tool that empowers you to take control of your health and well-being. It's a roadmap to achieving your best self while respecting your individuality and ethical boundaries. In the next sections, we will guide you through the process of creating a personalized biohacking plan, assessing your current state, selecting biohacking techniques, monitoring and tracking progress, and staying committed and adaptable.

Setting Clear and Specific Goals

Setting clear and specific goals is the foundational step in creating a personal biohacking plan. Your goals act as the guiding stars, directing your efforts and measuring your progress. In this section, we explore the importance of setting clear and specific biohacking goals:

Clarity and Direction:

- Clear and specific goals provide you with a sense of purpose and direction. Instead of vague aspirations like "being healthier," they define exactly what you aim to achieve, such as reducing cholesterol levels or increasing energy levels.

Motivation:

- Specific goals can be motivating. When you have a precise target in mind, it's easier to visualize your success, and this visualization can boost your motivation.

Measurable Progress:

- Specific goals are measurable. This means you can track your progress objectively. You'll know when you've achieved your goal because it's clearly defined.

Focus and Prioritization:

- Clear goals help you focus your biohacking efforts. They act as a filter, helping you decide which strategies and interventions are most relevant to your objectives.

Adaptation and Feedback:

- Well-defined goals allow you to adapt your plan as needed. If you're not making progress toward your goal, you can assess and adjust your strategies.

Consistency:

- Specific goals encourage consistency. When you know exactly what you're working towards, you're more likely to stick to your biohacking routines.

Ethical Considerations:

- Ensure that your goals are ethically sound and in alignment with your values. It's essential to pursue your objectives in a manner that respects your well-being and that of others.

In the following sections, we will guide you through the process of creating specific biohacking goals. We'll help you articulate your goals in a way that makes them clear, measurable, and aligned with your biohacking journey. Remember that your goals are personal to you, and the best goals are those that resonate with your aspirations and values.

Assessing Your Current State

Before you embark on your biohacking journey, it's crucial to assess your current state. This assessment serves as a baseline for measuring progress and tailoring your biohacking plan to your unique needs. In this section, we explore the process of assessing your current state:

Health Evaluation:

- Start by assessing your current health status. This includes physical health, mental well-being, and emotional balance. Take note of any existing medical conditions, medications, or chronic health issues.

Lifestyle Analysis:

- Analyze your current lifestyle, including dietary habits, exercise routines, sleep patterns, and stress levels. Recognize the areas where you are excelling and the ones that need improvement.

Goals Alignment:

- Consider how your current state aligns with your biohacking goals. Are there aspects of your life that are already in harmony with your objectives? Identify any discrepancies that may require adjustment.

Bioindicators and Metrics:

- Explore the use of bioindicators and metrics to gain deeper insights into your body's functioning. Metrics like blood pressure, cholesterol levels, and body composition can provide valuable data for tracking progress.

Psychological Evaluation:

- Evaluate your mental and emotional well-being. Consider factors like stress, anxiety, sleep quality, and cognitive performance. Understanding your psychological state is integral to your biohacking plan.

Biofeedback:

- Biofeedback devices can help provide real-time data on various aspects of your health, including heart rate variability, brainwave patterns, and stress levels. Consider using such tools to gather objective information.

Consultation:

- If needed, consult with healthcare professionals, nutritionists, or fitness experts to get a comprehensive assessment of your current health and well-being. Their insights can guide your biohacking journey.

Assessing your current state is a critical step that informs the creation of your personalized biohacking plan. It allows you to set realistic goals, track your progress effectively, and tailor your biohacking strategies to address your specific needs.

In the following sections, we will delve into the process of selecting biohacking techniques and monitoring and tracking your progress. These elements, along with your assessed current state, will help shape your biohacking journey.

If you'd like to continue with the next section or have any other specific requests, please feel free to let me know.

Selecting Biohacking Techniques

Once you have assessed your current state, the next crucial step in creating your personalized biohacking plan is selecting the appropriate biohacking techniques. Biohacking encompasses a wide range of practices, and choosing the right ones tailored to your needs is essential. In this section, we explore the process of selecting biohacking techniques:

Goal Alignment:

- Ensure that the techniques you select align with your biohacking goals. Whether your focus is on improving physical fitness, cognitive performance, or stress reduction, choose techniques that directly contribute to your objectives.

Research and Education:

- Take the time to research and educate yourself about different biohacking methods. Understand the science behind each technique and its potential benefits. Stay informed about the latest developments in the field.

Individual Needs:

- Consider your unique needs and preferences. Biohacking is a highly personalized journey, and what works for one person may not work for another. Choose techniques that resonate with your lifestyle and values.

Prioritization:

- Prioritize the techniques that address the areas where you need the most improvement. If, for example, you're dealing with sleep issues, prioritize biohacking techniques related to optimizing sleep quality.

Safety and Ethical Considerations:

- Ensure that the techniques you choose are safe and ethical. Biohacking should enhance your well-being without compromising your health or values. Avoid practices that may pose risks or ethical dilemmas.

Experimentation:

- Be open to experimentation. Biohacking often involves trial and error to discover what works best for you. Start with a manageable number of techniques and gradually incorporate new ones as you progress.

Consultation:

- If you're uncertain about which techniques to choose, seek advice from experienced biohackers, healthcare professionals, or experts in the field. They can provide valuable insights and recommendations.

Personalized Plan:

- Ultimately, your biohacking plan should be a tailored combination of techniques that suit your goals, align with your current state, and resonate with your preferences. A well-rounded approach can lead to holistic improvements.

By selecting biohacking techniques thoughtfully and customizing your plan, you set the stage for a more effective and rewarding biohacking journey. The techniques you choose should be in harmony with your goals and help you work towards becoming the best version of yourself.

In the following sections, we will explore the process of monitoring and tracking your progress and staying committed and adaptable in your biohacking journey.

Monitoring and Tracking Progress

Monitoring and tracking your progress are vital aspects of any biohacking journey. These activities provide you with valuable insights, enabling you to assess the effectiveness of your chosen techniques and make informed adjustments. In this section, we will explore the process of monitoring and tracking your biohacking progress:

Setting Clear Metrics and Benchmarks:

- Before you start monitoring, establish clear and measurable metrics and benchmarks. Define specific parameters that align with your biohacking goals. These could include factors like improved sleep quality, increased cognitive performance, or reduced stress levels.

Regular Data Collection:

- Consistently collect data related to your biohacking practices. This data may include information about your sleep patterns, dietary choices, exercise routines, cognitive performance, and any other relevant factors. Use tools like biofeedback devices, apps, or journals to record this data.

Data Analysis and Trend Identification:

- Regularly analyze the data you've collected. Look for trends and patterns that reveal the impact of your biohacking techniques. Identify which practices are contributing positively to your goals and which may need adjustments.

Making Informed Adjustments:

- Based on your data analysis, be prepared to make informed adjustments to your biohacking plan. If a particular technique is not delivering the desired results, consider modifying it or exploring alternative methods. Conversely, if you find a practice that yields significant improvements, continue to prioritize it.

Maintaining Motivation and Persistence:

- Biohacking is a journey that requires motivation and persistence. Track your progress not only to measure success but also to stay motivated. Seeing tangible improvements can boost your commitment to your biohacking plan.

Adaptability:

- Remain adaptable in your approach. As you gather more data and insights, your goals and priorities may evolve. Be open to adapting your plan to align with your changing needs and aspirations.

Monitoring and tracking your biohacking progress empower you to make evidence-based decisions that lead to positive outcomes. It ensures that you remain on the right path to achieving your goals and optimizing your health and well-being.

In the upcoming section, we will delve into strategies for overcoming common biohacking challenges.

Staying Committed and Adapting

Staying committed to your biohacking journey is essential for long-term success. It's a dynamic process that requires dedication and the ability to adapt as you learn more about your body and your goals. In this section, we'll explore the keys to maintaining commitment and adaptability in your biohacking endeavors:

Goal Reassessment:

- Periodically reassess your biohacking goals. As you make progress and gather more data, your objectives may change. Ensure that your goals remain aligned with your evolving aspirations for health, performance, and well-being.

Maintaining Consistency:

- Consistency is a cornerstone of effective biohacking. Stay consistent with your chosen techniques and routines to observe reliable results. Track your daily and weekly practices to ensure you're not deviating from your plan.

Seeking Support:

- Biohacking can be a solitary journey, but it's beneficial to seek support and guidance. Connect with communities, online forums, or mentors who can offer insights and motivation. Sharing experiences and knowledge with others can help keep you on track.

Self-Care and Recovery:

- Don't overlook the importance of self-care and recovery. Overextending yourself can lead to burnout and hinder your commitment. Ensure you prioritize rest, relaxation, and stress management as part of your biohacking plan.

Adapting to Challenges:

- Challenges are an inherent part of biohacking. As they arise, view them as opportunities for growth and adaptation. Learn from setbacks and use them to refine your approach.

Celebrate Achievements:

- Recognize and celebrate your achievements, no matter how small they may seem. Acknowledging progress and milestones along the way can boost your commitment and enthusiasm.

Periodic Assessments:

- Conduct periodic assessments of your biohacking plan. Analyze your progress, identify areas that need improvement, and make necessary adjustments to ensure you stay on track.

Maintaining commitment while staying adaptable is a delicate balance. By regularly reviewing your goals, maintaining consistency, seeking support, practicing self-care, and celebrating achievements, you can navigate the challenges and setbacks that may arise in your biohacking journey.

In the next section, we'll explore the process of monitoring and evaluating changes in your biohacking practices.

Chapter 12: Monitoring and Evaluation Process: Measuring and Assessing Changes

The Significance of Monitoring and Evaluation

Monitoring and evaluation are integral aspects of your biohacking journey. They provide a structured approach to assess the effectiveness of your strategies, make informed decisions, and optimize your path to improved health and performance.

Key Benefits of Monitoring and Evaluation:

1. Data-Driven Decisions: Monitoring and collecting data allow you to make evidence-based decisions about the effectiveness of your biohacking techniques. It's the foundation for informed adjustments.

2. Goal Tracking: You can measure your progress toward achieving your biohacking goals. This helps ensure you're on the right path and adjust your strategies as necessary.

3. Identification of Trends: Over time, you can identify trends in your data. For instance, you may notice how changes in nutrition or exercise impact your well-being. This knowledge can lead to more effective customization of your approach.

4. Prevention and Early Intervention: By tracking relevant metrics, you can identify issues or imbalances early, potentially preventing more significant health problems. For example, monitoring sleep patterns may help you address insomnia before it becomes chronic.

5. Motivation and Accountability: Seeing improvements or changes in your data can be motivating. It holds you accountable to your biohacking journey and keeps you engaged in the process.

6. Customization: Monitoring allows for customization. You can tailor your biohacking techniques based on your individual responses, maximizing their impact.

Data to Monitor:

- Depending on your biohacking objectives, the data you monitor can vary. Common metrics include sleep patterns, nutrition intake, exercise performance, mood, cognitive function, and physical health indicators like blood pressure, heart rate, and body composition.

Monitoring Tools:

- Utilize various tools and devices to collect data, such as fitness trackers, smart scales, mood journals, and specialized biohacking apps. These tools simplify the process of data collection and analysis.

Frequency of Monitoring:

- The frequency of monitoring depends on your goals and the specific metrics you're tracking. Some aspects, like sleep, may require daily tracking, while others can be assessed weekly or monthly.

Monitoring and evaluation are not only essential for assessing progress but also for refining your biohacking plan to achieve optimal results. In the next sections, we'll delve deeper into setting clear metrics and benchmarks, regular data collection, data analysis, making informed adjustments, and maintaining motivation and persistence in your biohacking journey.

Setting Clear Metrics and Benchmarks

In your biohacking journey, setting clear metrics and benchmarks is vital for achieving your desired results. These metrics serve as the yardsticks against which you can measure your progress and the effectiveness of your biohacking strategies.

Importance of Clear Metrics and Benchmarks:

1. Goal Clarity: Clear metrics provide a precise definition of your biohacking goals. Whether you aim to improve sleep quality, enhance cognitive performance, or optimize your physical fitness, having specific metrics makes your objectives concrete.

2. Progress Tracking: Benchmarks help you monitor your progress over time. By comparing your current status to these benchmarks, you can see how far you've come and make necessary adjustments.

3. Objective Decision-Making: When you have established metrics, you can make informed decisions about which biohacking techniques are working and which ones need modification. This prevents guesswork and ensures evidence-based choices.

4. Motivation: Achieving incremental milestones can be motivating. It gives you a sense of accomplishment and encourages you to stay committed to your biohacking journey.

Creating Effective Metrics:

1. Specificity: Metrics should be specific and well-defined. For instance, if you want to improve sleep, a specific metric could be "average nightly sleep duration in hours."

2. Measurability: Ensure that you can measure the chosen metrics accurately. This may require the use of tracking tools or devices, such as sleep trackers or heart rate monitors.

3. Relevance: The metrics should align with your biohacking goals. They should directly reflect the aspects of your health and performance that you aim to enhance.

4. Realism: Set benchmarks that are realistic and attainable. While ambitious goals are good, they should also be within reach to maintain motivation.

5. Time Frame: Establish a timeframe for achieving your benchmarks. For example, you may aim to improve your running speed by 10% in three months.

Examples of Metrics and Benchmarks:

- Sleep Improvement: Achieve an average of 7.5 hours of high-quality sleep per night within three months.

- Cognitive Enhancement: Enhance cognitive performance by achieving a 15% improvement in memory test scores within six months.

- Physical Fitness: Increase muscle mass by 5% and reduce body fat by 3% in four months.

Regularly Reviewing and Updating Metrics:

As you progress in your biohacking journey, it's important to periodically review and update your metrics and benchmarks. What's attainable or relevant may change, and your goals may evolve. This adaptability ensures that your biohacking plan remains effective and aligned with your aspirations.

In the following sections, we'll explore the importance of regular data collection, data analysis, making informed adjustments, and maintaining motivation and persistence in your biohacking journey.

Regular Data Collection

Regular data collection is a cornerstone of effective biohacking. It involves the systematic gathering of information related to your biohacking goals and metrics. This data serves as the basis for evaluating your progress and making informed adjustments to your biohacking strategies.

The Importance of Regular Data Collection:

1. Data-Driven Decisions: Collecting data provides you with objective insights into how your body and mind are responding to biohacking techniques. This data empowers you to make informed decisions regarding which strategies are working and which require modification.

2. Progress Monitoring: Data collection allows you to track your progress over time. By regularly documenting relevant metrics, you can observe trends, identify patterns, and gauge the effectiveness of your biohacking efforts.

3. Early Problem Detection: Regular data collection can help you identify issues or setbacks early on. This enables you to address problems promptly, minimizing the potential for long-term setbacks.

4. Feedback Loop: A feedback loop is established through data collection. As you observe how your body responds to specific biohacking interventions, you can fine-tune your strategies to achieve optimal results.

Effective Data Collection Practices:

1. Consistency: Ensure that data collection is a routine part of your biohacking journey. Consistency is key in detecting trends and changes.

2. Use of Tools: Utilize appropriate tools and technologies to collect data accurately. This may include fitness trackers, apps for nutrition tracking, or wearables that monitor physiological parameters.

3. Data Storage: Safely store your data, either digitally or in a dedicated notebook. This allows you to revisit and analyze your progress over time.

4. Real-Time Monitoring: In some cases, real-time data monitoring can be particularly beneficial. For example, continuous glucose monitoring provides immediate insights into how different foods affect your blood sugar levels.

Types of Data to Collect:

The specific data you collect depends on your biohacking goals and the associated metrics. Common types of data include:

- **Sleep Patterns:** Data on your sleep duration, quality, and disruptions.

- **Nutrition:** Records of your dietary intake, macronutrient ratios, and micronutrient consumption.

- **Physical Activity:** Information on your exercise routines, intensity, and duration.

- **Biometric Data:** Physiological parameters such as heart rate, blood pressure, and body composition.

- **Cognitive Performance:** Data on memory, focus, and mental clarity.

- **Stress Levels:** Measurements of stress responses through heart rate variability or self-reporting.

Review and Analysis:

Regularly reviewing and analyzing the data you collect is crucial. Look for trends, patterns, and correlations. Identify what works and what doesn't, and be open to making necessary adjustments to your biohacking strategies based on this analysis.

In the subsequent sections, we will delve into data analysis, making informed adjustments, and maintaining motivation and persistence in your biohacking journey. If you'd like to proceed with a specific subsection or have any other requests, please let me know.

Data Analysis and Trend Identification

Effective data analysis and trend identification are essential components of successful biohacking. These processes enable you to gain insights from the data you've collected, understand how your body responds to various interventions, and refine your biohacking strategies accordingly.

Data Analysis Process:

1. Data Organization: Begin by organizing your data systematically. Create a clear structure for storing and accessing the information you've collected. This organization ensures that you can easily retrieve and review your data when needed.

2. Data Visualization: Visual representations of data, such as graphs and charts, are powerful tools for understanding trends. Use software or apps to create visualizations that highlight patterns and changes over time.

3. Correlation Assessment: Look for correlations between different variables. For example, you may analyze whether specific dietary changes are correlated with improvements in sleep quality or cognitive performance. Identifying correlations can guide your biohacking decisions.

4. Trend Identification: One of the primary goals of data analysis is to identify trends. Trends represent consistent patterns in your data. These patterns can be positive (indicating improvements) or negative (indicating setbacks). For example, you might notice that your sleep duration improves as you increase your physical activity levels.

Trend Identification and Utilization:

1. Positive Trends: If you identify positive trends, such as improved sleep quality or increased cognitive performance, consider reinforcing the strategies that led to these improvements. Positive trends indicate that certain biohacking interventions are effective for you.

2. Negative Trends: Negative trends, like deteriorating sleep patterns or declining physical fitness, signal that adjustments are needed. Use the data to pinpoint the specific factors contributing to these negative trends, and modify your biohacking approaches accordingly.

3. Goal Alignment: Assess trends in relation to your biohacking goals. If the identified trends align with your desired outcomes, you're on the right track. If they don't align, it's time to reevaluate your strategies.

4. Regular Review: Data analysis should be an ongoing process. Regularly review your data and trends to track your progress, make informed decisions, and adapt your biohacking plan to your evolving needs and goals.

In the subsequent sections, we will cover making informed adjustments based on data analysis, maintaining motivation and persistence, and overcoming common biohacking challenges.

Making Informed Adjustments

Once you've conducted a thorough data analysis and identified trends in your biohacking journey, the next crucial step is to make informed adjustments. Adjustments are essential for fine-tuning your biohacking techniques to achieve your goals. Here's a guide on how to make informed adjustments:

Evaluate Trends and Outcomes:

1. Positive Trends: If you've identified positive trends, it's a clear indication that certain aspects of your biohacking strategies are working effectively. Evaluate what specific interventions led to these positive changes, such as dietary modifications, exercise routines, or sleep quality improvements.

2. Negative Trends: Negative trends, such as declining sleep quality or decreased mental clarity, are indicators that certain elements of your biohacking plan may need revision. Carefully assess what factors could be contributing to these negative changes.

Targeted Adjustments:

3. Specific Changes: Based on your evaluation, consider making targeted changes. If certain dietary habits positively influenced your cognitive performance, try to refine and optimize those habits. Conversely, if you found that late-night screen time affected your sleep negatively, plan adjustments to reduce this issue.

4. Gradual Modifications: Avoid making abrupt or extreme changes. Gradual modifications allow your body to adapt more smoothly and help you gauge their impact over time. For instance, if you want to change your exercise routine, introduce the adjustments progressively.

Goal Alignment:

5. Align with Your Goals: Ensure that all adjustments align with your biohacking objectives. Your goals provide the compass for your journey. If an adjustment doesn't contribute to achieving your goals, reconsider its relevance.

6. Realistic Expectations: Understand that achieving your biohacking goals may take time. Be patient and maintain realistic expectations. Rome wasn't built in a day, and lasting, positive changes may require consistent effort.

Monitoring and Tracking:

7. Continued Data Collection: Continue monitoring and tracking your progress, even after making adjustments. This ongoing process enables you to assess the effectiveness of your modifications and make further adjustments as necessary.

8. Iteration: Biohacking is an iterative process. Expect to revisit and adjust your strategies regularly as your body and goals evolve.

Seek Professional Guidance:

9. Consultation: In some cases, especially when dealing with complex health issues or extreme goals, consider consulting a healthcare professional or a biohacking expert. Their expertise can provide valuable insights and guidance.

Remember that the key to successful biohacking is adaptability and continuous learning. Making informed adjustments based on data analysis is an integral part of the biohacking journey. In the following sections, we'll cover maintaining motivation and persistence, overcoming common biohacking challenges, and progress tracking.

Maintaining Motivation and Persistence

Maintaining motivation and persistence are vital components of a successful biohacking journey. Biohacking, like any long-term endeavor, comes with its share of challenges. Here's how to stay motivated and persistent:

Set Clear and Realistic Goals:

1. Goal Clarity: Ensure your biohacking goals are specific, measurable, attainable, relevant, and time-bound (SMART). Clearly defined goals provide a sense of purpose and direction.

2. Subgoals: Divide larger goals into smaller, achievable subgoals. Each milestone you reach reinforces motivation.

Positive Reinforcement:

3. Celebrate Achievements: Acknowledge and celebrate your accomplishments, no matter how small. Positive reinforcement boosts motivation.

4. Visualize Success: Imagine the positive outcomes of reaching your biohacking goals. Visualization can be a powerful motivational tool.

Progress Tracking:

5. Data and Trends: Regularly review your data and the trends you've identified. Seeing the results of your efforts can be a strong motivator.

6. Monitoring Progress: Continue tracking your biohacking journey and take note of improvements. Knowing that you're making progress can help you stay motivated.

Education and Learning:

7. Stay Informed: Continuously educate yourself about biohacking, health, and performance improvement. Learning new strategies and understanding the science behind biohacking can be motivating.

8. Experimentation: Treat biohacking as an ongoing experiment. The curiosity to see how your body responds to different interventions can be exciting.

Accountability and Support:

9. Accountability Partners: Consider having an accountability partner or joining a biohacking community. Sharing your progress and challenges with others can help you stay on track.

10. Professional Guidance: If needed, consult with healthcare professionals or biohacking experts. Their support and guidance can be invaluable.

Mindset and Resilience:

11. Positive Mindset: Cultivate a growth mindset and understand that setbacks are a part of the journey. Use them as opportunities to learn and grow.

12. Resilience: Develop resilience to bounce back from challenges. Biohacking often involves experimentation, and not every attempt will yield immediate results.

Consistency and Patience:

13. Routine and Consistency: Establish a biohacking routine that you can maintain. Consistency is key for long-term success.

14. Patience: Understand that biohacking is a gradual process. Some changes may take time to manifest.

Remember that maintaining motivation and persistence in biohacking is about creating a sustainable and enjoyable journey. The ability to adapt, stay resilient, and keep working towards your goals will lead to better results over time.

Chapter 13: Overcoming Barriers and Challenges

Recognizing Common Biohacking Challenges

Biohacking is a journey of self-improvement and optimization, but like any journey, it comes with its share of challenges. To overcome these challenges, it's essential to first recognize them. Here are some common biohacking challenges you might encounter:

1. Lack of Consistency and Motivation:

- Maintaining consistency in your biohacking practices can be challenging. Motivation may wane over time, making it difficult to stick to your routines.

2. Information Overload and Confusion:

- The abundance of information on biohacking can lead to confusion. Sorting through the wealth of advice and strategies can be overwhelming.

3. Time Constraints:

- Balancing biohacking with a busy schedule can be tough. Finding time for meal preparation, exercise, and other biohacking activities might seem challenging.

4. Financial Limitations:

- Some biohacking interventions and tools can be costly. Financial constraints may limit your options.

5. Overcoming Plateaus and Setbacks:

- It's common to face plateaus in your progress or even experience setbacks. These moments can be disheartening and demotivating.

6. Social and Peer Pressure:

- Social situations and peer pressure can influence your biohacking journey. Staying committed to your goals in the face of social norms can be a challenge.

7. Psychological Barriers:

- Your mental state and psychological barriers, such as fear of failure or self-doubt, can hinder your biohacking progress.

Recognizing these challenges is the first step in addressing them effectively. In the following subsections, we'll delve into strategies and techniques to overcome these challenges and navigate your biohacking journey successfully.

Lack of Consistency and Motivation

Maintaining consistency and staying motivated are pivotal challenges that many individuals encounter when embarking on a biohacking journey. The initial excitement and determination can wane over time, making it challenging to adhere to biohacking practices. Here are some strategies to combat this issue:

1. Set Clear Goals: Begin by establishing well-defined and achievable goals for your biohacking journey. Having clear objectives provides a sense of purpose and motivation. Make these goals specific, measurable, and time-bound (SMART) to track your progress effectively.

2. Create a Routine: Consistency often thrives on routine. Develop a daily or weekly schedule that incorporates your biohacking activities. This schedule should align with your goals and accommodate your daily life.

3. Track Your Progress: Regularly monitor and record your progress. This not only helps in assessing how far you've come but also acts as a motivating factor. Seeing improvements can reignite your commitment.

4. Find an Accountability Partner: Consider teaming up with a friend or a community that shares your interest in biohacking. Having someone to hold you accountable and share the journey can help maintain motivation.

5. Celebrate Small Wins: Acknowledge and celebrate your small achievements along the way. Recognizing progress, no matter how minor, boosts motivation. This can be as simple as a pat on the back or a small treat.

6. Stay Informed: Continuously educate yourself about biohacking techniques and their benefits. Learning new things and understanding the science behind biohacking can keep your interest alive.

7. Adapt and Experiment: Biohacking is a flexible journey. Don't be afraid to experiment with new strategies and adapt your approach as you learn. The element of novelty can inject enthusiasm into your biohacking practices.

8. Mindset and Visualization: Cultivate a positive mindset and use visualization techniques. Envision the positive changes and improvements you'll achieve through biohacking. A positive outlook can drive consistency.

9. Rewards and Incentives: Create a system of rewards or incentives for reaching milestones. Knowing that a reward awaits you can be a powerful motivator.

Remember that motivation can fluctuate, and it's normal to face periods of lower enthusiasm. By incorporating these strategies, you can maintain consistency and overcome motivational slumps during your biohacking journey.

Information Overload and Confusion aps and Tree Diagrams

Biohacking is a field with a wealth of information, techniques, and tools, which can sometimes lead to information overload and confusion. Navigating through the vast sea of biohacking knowledge can be challenging. Here are some strategies to help you overcome information overload and confusion:

1. Start with the Basics: Begin your biohacking journey by focusing on fundamental principles and practices. Gradually delve into more complex techniques as you gain experience and confidence.

2. Set Priorities: Identify specific areas of biohacking that align with your goals. Prioritize your efforts on the techniques and practices that are most relevant to your objectives.

3. Seek Reliable Sources: Ensure that you're gathering information from reputable and evidence-based sources. Be critical of claims that lack scientific backing.

4. Experiment Gradually: Avoid the temptation to try every biohacking method simultaneously. Instead, introduce new techniques one at a time, assess their impact, and adjust accordingly.

5. Consult Experts: If you're feeling overwhelmed, consider seeking guidance from experienced biohackers or health professionals. They can provide tailored advice and help you avoid confusion.

6. Keep Records: Maintain a detailed record of your biohacking activities, including the techniques you're trying, their effects, and any challenges you face. This helps in tracking what works best for you.

7. Regularly Review Your Goals: Periodically revisit your biohacking goals and adjust your practices accordingly. This ensures that you're on the right path and not wasting efforts on irrelevant techniques.

8. Avoid Quick Fixes: Be cautious of biohacking solutions that promise rapid results. True biohacking is often a gradual and long-term process that requires consistency.

9. Share and Connect: Join biohacking communities or forums where you can share experiences and gain insights from others who are on similar journeys. This can help reduce confusion through shared knowledge.

10. Practice Critical Thinking: Develop your critical thinking skills to discern between well-founded biohacking methods and pseudoscientific claims. Skepticism is a valuable tool in this field.

Information overload and confusion are common challenges, especially for newcomers to biohacking. By adopting these strategies, you can streamline your biohacking journey, make informed choices, and reduce the risk of becoming overwhelmed by excessive information.

Time Constraints

One of the most common barriers to biohacking is the limitation of time. Modern life often demands our attention and commitment to various responsibilities, leaving little room for extensive biohacking endeavors. However, with effective time management and prioritization, you can still integrate biohacking into your life. Here's how to address time constraints:

1. Set Realistic Expectations: Understand that biohacking doesn't always require large time commitments. Begin with small, manageable changes that fit your schedule.

2. Prioritize Your Health: Recognize that investing time in your health and well-being is an essential aspect of biohacking. Consider it a long-term commitment that pays off in various aspects of your life.

3. Time Blocking: Allocate specific time slots in your daily or weekly schedule for biohacking activities. Consistency is often more important than the duration of individual sessions.

4. Multitasking: Combine biohacking practices with other activities when possible. For instance, practice deep breathing or mindfulness during your daily commute or perform stretching exercises during short breaks.

5. Streamline Your Routine: Look for ways to optimize your daily routine. For example, prepare healthy meals in advance, ensuring you have nutritious options readily available.

6. Sleep Optimization: Prioritize quality sleep, as it enhances overall efficiency and productivity, potentially saving time during the day.

7. Leverage Technology: Use biohacking apps and wearable devices to monitor and track your progress. These tools can save time by providing valuable insights with minimal effort.

8. Delegate Tasks: Whenever possible, delegate non-essential tasks to free up time for biohacking. It could be outsourcing certain responsibilities or seeking help from family and friends.

9. Set Clear Goals: Focus on biohacking techniques that align with your specific goals. This prevents time wastage on irrelevant practices.

10. Batching: Group similar biohacking activities together. For instance, dedicate a specific day for meal preparation and planning for the week.

11. Efficient Workouts: If exercise is a part of your biohacking regimen, consider high-intensity workouts that deliver benefits in shorter time frames.

12. Regular Assessments: Periodically evaluate your biohacking practices to ensure they remain time-efficient and effective.

13. Stress Management: Implement stress-reduction techniques as stress can consume a significant portion of your time and energy.

14. Flexible Approach: Be adaptable in your biohacking journey. If certain techniques become too time-consuming, find alternative practices that are more sustainable within your schedule.

Time constraints are a common challenge, but with strategic planning and commitment, biohacking can be integrated into even the busiest of lifestyles. The key is to make the most of the time you have available and focus on practices that offer the greatest benefits in the shortest time.

Financial Limitations

Biohacking, like many pursuits, can involve expenses for equipment, supplements, and specialized services. However, it's essential to understand that effective biohacking doesn't always require significant financial investments. Here's how to address financial limitations and still engage in biohacking practices:

1. Prioritize Essentials: Focus on biohacking practices that don't strain your budget. Basic practices like improving sleep quality, eating nutritious whole foods, and regular physical activity can be accomplished without substantial costs.

2. Plan Your Budget: Allocate a specific budget for biohacking activities. This ensures you're not overspending while still pursuing your goals.

3. DIY Approaches: Many biohacking practices can be done using do-it-yourself (DIY) methods. For example, creating a home workout routine, practicing mindfulness without expensive apps, or growing your own organic herbs.

4. Open-Source Resources: Explore free or open-source resources for biohacking information, such as online articles, forums, and communities. Many biohackers share their knowledge and experiences without charge.

5. Choose Cost-Effective Supplements: If you're considering supplements, prioritize those that offer the most benefits for your specific goals. Don't overspend on unnecessary products.

6. Discounts and Sales: Keep an eye out for discounts, promotions, and sales on biohacking equipment, supplements, and tools. Online retailers often offer deals.

7. Buy Secondhand: Consider purchasing used or secondhand biohacking equipment, especially for items like exercise gear or wearable devices.

8. Subscription Services: Some biohacking services, such as genetic testing or meal delivery, offer subscription plans that may be more cost-effective over time.

9. Consult Experts Selectively: While consulting with professionals can be beneficial, it's not always necessary. Choose expert services selectively when the potential benefits outweigh the costs.

10. Trade and Barter: Explore the possibility of trading services or goods with others who share your biohacking interests. This can be a cost-effective way to access specialized resources.

11. Government Programs: Investigate whether government or community programs offer support for health and wellness initiatives. Some regions have resources available for free or at reduced costs.

12. Educate Yourself: Invest time in learning about biohacking principles and techniques. Knowledge can be a powerful tool for maximizing benefits without heavy financial investments.

13. Long-Term View: Consider the long-term savings associated with biohacking. By improving your health and well-being, you may reduce healthcare costs in the future.

Remember that biohacking doesn't require significant financial resources. With a practical approach, you can make progress toward your biohacking goals while being mindful of your budget. Prioritize practices that align with your goals and explore cost-effective solutions that suit your needs.

Overcoming Plateaus and Setbacks

Biohacking is a journey filled with ups and downs. Plateaus and setbacks are natural occurrences on this path. However, how you deal with them can significantly impact your progress. Here's how to overcome these challenges:

1. Reevaluate Your Approach: When you hit a plateau or face a setback, it's essential to reevaluate your biohacking practices. Assess whether what worked in the past is still effective or if changes are needed.

2. Set New Goals: Adjust your goals to reflect your current circumstances. Sometimes, plateauing occurs because you've reached your initial objectives. Setting new, challenging goals can reignite your motivation.

3. Vary Your Practices: Change your routines, exercises, or biohacking techniques. Adding variety to your practices can help break through plateaus and overcome boredom.

4. Be Patient: Plateaus can be frustrating, but remember that progress is not always linear. It may take some time before you notice improvements again. Patience is key.

5. Seek Support: Don't hesitate to reach out to a community of biohackers or a mentor. Sharing your experiences and receiving feedback can provide valuable insights and motivation.

6. Consult a Professional: If you're facing a particularly challenging setback, consider consulting a healthcare professional or specialist. They can help identify underlying issues and tailor solutions to your specific needs.

7. Track Your Data: Continue monitoring your progress and gather data to pinpoint areas that need improvement. Data analysis can help you identify patterns and make informed decisions.

8. Mindset Matters: Approach plateaus with a growth mindset. View them as opportunities for learning and adapting, rather than failures.

9. Recharge Your Motivation: Take a break if needed. Sometimes, stepping away from your biohacking practices for a short time can reignite your motivation and help you return with a fresh perspective.

10. Review Your Lifestyle: Consider factors outside of your biohacking practices that may be affecting your progress. Stress, sleep quality, and other lifestyle elements play a significant role in your overall well-being.

11. Stay Consistent: Even during plateaus, it's essential to maintain consistency in your practices. Consistency can help you break through the plateau when the time is right.

12. Celebrate Small Wins: Acknowledge and celebrate even the smallest achievements. This positive reinforcement can keep you motivated during challenging times.

13. Long-Term Perspective: Remember that biohacking is a long-term endeavor. Plateaus and setbacks are part of the journey, and they don't define your ultimate success.

Biohacking is a dynamic process, and there will be phases of rapid progress and periods of stagnation. Overcoming plateaus and setbacks is a testament to your commitment and adaptability. By approaching these challenges with resilience and the willingness to adjust your strategies, you can continue making positive changes to your well-being.

Social and Peer Pressure

One of the often-overlooked challenges in the world of biohacking is the influence of social and peer pressure. When embarking on a journey to improve your health and well-being through biohacking, it's common to encounter individuals who may not fully understand or support your choices. Here's how to navigate social and peer pressure effectively:

1. Educate and Communicate: Take the time to explain the concept of biohacking and its benefits to your friends and family. Knowledge can often dispel misconceptions and create a more supportive environment.

2. Find Like-Minded Communities: Seek out biohacking communities, either in person or online, where you can connect with individuals who share similar goals and values. Surrounding yourself with like-minded people can provide a strong support system.

3. Set Boundaries: Politely but firmly establish boundaries with those who may question or undermine your biohacking practices. Let them know that your choices are based on your personal goals and preferences.

4. Lead by Example: Demonstrating the positive effects of biohacking in your own life can be a powerful way to influence those around you. When your friends and family witness your improvements in health, focus, and well-being, they may become more open to the idea.

5. Respect Differences: Understand that not everyone will be interested in biohacking, and that's okay. Respect their choices just as you would like them to respect yours. Encourage open dialogue rather than confrontation.

6. Stay Confident: Confidence in your biohacking journey can be a shield against external pressures. Be sure of your choices, and remember that you are making decisions that align with your goals and values.

7. Focus on Your Goals: Keep your objectives in mind and remind yourself of why you started biohacking in the first place. When your goals are clear and important to you, it becomes easier to resist external pressures.

8. Seek Supportive Friends: Surround yourself with friends and acquaintances who understand and respect your biohacking journey. Sharing your experiences with individuals who support your choices can be motivating.

9. Use Social Media Wisely: Social media can be a valuable tool for connecting with like-minded individuals and sharing your progress. Use it as a platform to inspire and be inspired.

10. Be Patient: It may take time for those around you to fully embrace your biohacking practices. Be patient with their questions or concerns, and be open to addressing them when the opportunity arises.

11. Lead with Empathy: Remember that people may have concerns about your biohacking practices out of genuine care for your well-being. Approach conversations with empathy and understanding.

While social and peer pressure can present challenges, it's essential to remain true to your biohacking journey and make choices that align with your goals. Over time, as you continue to experience the benefits and improvements in your life, you may find that others become more open to understanding and supporting your path to better health and well-being.

Psychological Barriers

In the realm of biohacking, where the focus is on improving physical and mental well-being, overcoming psychological barriers is crucial. These barriers often stem from the mind and can be just as challenging as external obstacles. Here are some common psychological barriers biohackers may encounter and how to address them:

1. Self-Doubt: Many biohackers start their journey with a level of self-doubt. They question whether they can achieve the goals they've set for themselves. Overcoming self-doubt requires self-awareness and patience. Set realistic, achievable goals, and track your progress. Small successes build confidence over time.

2. Perfectionism: Striving for perfection in biohacking can be counterproductive. The fear of not doing everything perfectly can lead to anxiety and stress. Remember that biohacking is about continuous improvement, not perfection. Embrace the concept of gradual progress.

3. Impatience: Biohacking is a long-term endeavor, and the desire for immediate results can lead to frustration. Practice patience and recognize that changes may take time. Track your progress and celebrate small wins along the way.

4. Comparison: Comparing your biohacking journey to others can lead to feelings of inadequacy. It's important to remember that each person's journey is unique, and everyone starts from a different point. Focus on your own progress rather than comparing it to others.

5. Fear of Failure: The fear of failing at biohacking can be paralyzing. Remember that setbacks and failures are part of any journey. Embrace them as opportunities to learn and grow. Analyze what went wrong, make adjustments, and keep moving forward.

6. Lack of Motivation: Motivation can ebb and flow, and there will be days when you lack enthusiasm for your biohacking practices. To overcome this, establish a routine and make biohacking a habit. Find sources of inspiration, such as success stories or personal goals.

7. Negative Self-Talk: Negative self-talk can sabotage your biohacking efforts. Replace self-criticism with self-encouragement and positive affirmations. Focus on your accomplishments and acknowledge your strengths.

8. Stress and Anxiety: Biohacking can become stressful if not managed properly. Incorporate stress-reduction techniques, such as mindfulness, meditation, or deep breathing, into your routine. Addressing stress can improve overall well-being.

9. Overthinking: Overanalyzing biohacking techniques and data can lead to analysis paralysis. Keep it simple and choose a few key practices that align with your goals. Avoid getting lost in the details.

10. Burnout: Biohackers who push themselves too hard may experience burnout. Balance is essential. Make time for relaxation, leisure, and recovery to avoid burnout and maintain your commitment to biohacking.

11. Body Image Concerns: Biohacking isn't about achieving a particular body image. It's about optimizing your health and performance. Avoid falling into the trap of extreme dieting or exercise solely for aesthetic purposes.

Addressing these psychological barriers is as important as addressing physical challenges. Recognize that overcoming these barriers is a process, and be compassionate with yourself as you work toward a healthier and more balanced life. Incorporate practices like self-care, self-reflection, and seeking support from friends and mentors to help you overcome these mental obstacles.

Chapter 14: Progress Tracking Notebook: Monitoring and Recording Development

As you embark on your biohacking journey, keeping a Progress Tracking Notebook is an invaluable tool for monitoring and recording your development. This notebook serves as a centralized hub for collecting data, insights, and observations related to your biohacking practices and their impact on your health and well-being.

14.1 The Importance of Progress Tracking

Monitoring your progress is essential for several reasons:

- **Accountability:** A Progress Tracking Notebook holds you accountable for the biohacking techniques you've committed to. It ensures you stick to your plan.

- **Data Collection:** It allows you to gather data related to your biohacking practices, including nutritional changes, exercise routines, sleep patterns, and other key aspects.

- **Trend Identification:** Over time, tracking your progress helps you identify trends and correlations between specific practices and improvements or setbacks.

- **Informed Adjustments:** When you have a detailed record of your biohacking journey, you can make informed adjustments. If something isn't working as expected, you can pinpoint the issue and modify your approach.

- **Motivation:** Looking back at your progress and seeing how far you've come can be a powerful motivator, helping you stay committed to your biohacking goals.

14.2 Setting Up Your Progress Tracking Notebook

Here's how to set up an effective Progress Tracking Notebook:

- **Choose a Notebook:** Opt for a dedicated notebook or journal. You can also use digital tools and apps for this purpose, depending on your preference.

- **Sections and Categories:** Create sections or categories within your notebook to organize your data. Consider sections for nutrition, exercise, sleep, stress management, and any other relevant biohacking aspects.

- **Data Entry:** Regularly update your notebook with data, observations, and insights. This can include details about your meals, exercise routines, sleep quality, stress levels, and any other biohacking activities.

- **Daily Entries:** Aim to make daily entries if possible. Recording your daily experiences and practices will provide a comprehensive view of your journey.

- **Include Metrics:** Incorporate relevant metrics, such as sleep duration, exercise intensity, dietary macronutrients, and subjective well-being scores. Metrics allow for more objective assessment.

- **Graphs and Charts:** Consider creating graphs or charts to visualize trends and changes in your data. This can be especially helpful for tracking progress over time.

14.3 Recording Development and Insights

In your Progress Tracking Notebook, record:

- **Successes:** Document the positive outcomes you've experienced as a result of your biohacking practices. Celebrate your achievements, whether they relate to physical performance, mental clarity, or overall well-being.

- **Setbacks:** Be honest about any setbacks or challenges you encounter. Identifying setbacks is the first step in addressing and overcoming them.

- **Insights:** Record personal insights and observations. This can include how specific dietary changes affect your energy levels, how certain exercises impact your mood, or how sleep quality influences your cognitive function.

- **Adjustments:** Note any adjustments you've made to your biohacking plan. Explain the reasons for these adjustments and the outcomes you hope to achieve.

14.4 Regular Review

Set aside time for regular reviews of your Progress Tracking Notebook. This could be weekly, monthly, or at intervals that suit your biohacking journey. During these reviews:

- **Analyze Trends**: Examine trends and patterns in your data. Look for correlations between specific practices and outcomes.

- **Evaluate Progress**: Assess your overall progress and whether you are moving closer to your biohacking goals.

- **Adapt Your Plan:** If necessary, adapt your biohacking plan based on the insights you've gathered from your tracking.

- Stay Motivated: Use your notebook as a source of motivation. Remind yourself of the progress you've made and the improvements in your health and well-being.

A Progress Tracking Notebook is a dynamic tool that evolves as you progress on your biohacking journey. It provides a structured way to collect and analyze data, ensuring that you stay on course and continue optimizing your life for the better. Remember that the insights you gain from your tracking will be instrumental in achieving your biohacking goals.

PART V
Your Journey to a Better Version of Yourself

Chapter 15: Embarking on Your Journey: Entering Change and Improvement

Embarking on a journey of change and self-improvement through biohacking is a remarkable decision. It signifies your commitment to enhancing your health, well-being, and overall quality of life. In this chapter, we will explore the essential steps to take as you begin your biohacking journey:

1. Clarify Your Goals: Clearly define the goals you want to achieve through biohacking. Whether it's better physical fitness, enhanced mental clarity, improved sleep, or other objectives, setting specific and achievable goals provides a roadmap for your journey.

2. Assess Your Starting Point: Take stock of your current health and well-being. This includes physical health, mental health, lifestyle, and habits. An honest assessment will help you identify areas that need improvement.

3. Research and Learn: Biohacking involves experimenting with various techniques and approaches. Invest time in research and learning about different biohacking methods, technologies, and practices. Knowledge is your best tool on this journey.

4. Seek Guidance: Consider consulting with experts, such as nutritionists, fitness trainers, and health professionals, to gain insights tailored to your needs and goals. Their guidance can be invaluable in creating a personalized biohacking plan.

5. Design Your Biohacking Plan: Create a personalized biohacking plan that aligns with your goals. This plan should include specific practices, dietary changes, exercise routines, and other biohacking techniques. Your plan should be adaptable and realistic.

6. Implement Gradual Changes: Avoid making drastic changes all at once. Instead, implement gradual, sustainable adjustments to your lifestyle. Slow and steady progress is more likely to lead to lasting results.

7. Record and Monitor Progress: Keeping a journal to document your biohacking journey is crucial. Track changes in your physical health, mental clarity, sleep quality, and overall well-being. This data will help you make informed adjustments.

8. Stay Consistent: Consistency is key in biohacking. Commit to your plan and practice your chosen biohacking methods regularly. Over time, consistency will yield significant improvements.

9. Stay Adaptable: Be prepared to adapt your biohacking plan as you gain experience and insights. What works for one person may not work for another, so flexibility and openness to change are essential.

10. Stay Patient: Biohacking is a long-term endeavor. It may take time to see significant changes, so practice patience and celebrate small milestones along the way.

11. Engage with the Biohacking Community: Biohacking is a rapidly evolving field, and there's a vibrant community of biohackers eager to share knowledge and experiences. Engage with this community to learn from others and find inspiration.

12. Practice Self-Care: Remember that biohacking is about optimizing your health and well-being. Incorporate self-care practices like stress management, relaxation, and mindfulness into your daily routine.

13. Maintain Balance: Balance is crucial in biohacking. Don't become obsessed with optimization to the point of neglecting other aspects of your life. Ensure you have a balanced approach to health and well-being.

Embarking on your biohacking journey is an exciting and transformative process. The journey itself is as important as the destination. By following these steps, you'll be well-prepared to make significant improvements in your life, optimize your health, and become the best version of yourself. Your biohacking journey is a personal adventure that will lead to meaningful change and self-discovery.

Chapter 16: Integration and Long-Term Implementation: Secrets to Sustaining Biohacking and Optimal Health

Embarking on a biohacking journey and making significant improvements in your health and well-being is a commendable achievement. However, sustaining the positive changes you've worked hard to attain requires a different set of strategies and a long-term perspective. In this chapter, we explore the secrets to integrating biohacking practices into your life and maintaining optimal health for the long run.

16.1 Embracing Biohacking as a Lifestyle

Biohacking is most effective when it becomes an integral part of your lifestyle. Instead of viewing it as a temporary fix or a short-term experiment, adopt it as a long-term commitment to your well-being. Here are some key aspects of embracing biohacking as a lifestyle:

- **Consistency:** Consistency is the bedrock of sustainable biohacking. Your practices should become daily routines or habits, just like brushing your teeth or eating meals.

- **Integration:** Integrate biohacking seamlessly into your life. This means that your biohacking activities should fit into your daily schedule and complement your existing commitments.

- **Mindset Shift:** Cultivate a biohacker's mindset. This involves viewing your body and mind as an ongoing project, always open to improvement. Embrace challenges and seek opportunities for optimization.

16.2 Long-Term Health vs. Quick Fixes

Many biohackers understand that achieving optimal health is a long-term endeavor. Instead of seeking quick fixes or short-term gains, they focus on long-term health goals. Here's how you can approach this perspective:

- **Avoiding Extreme Measures:** Extreme diets, intensive workouts, or other extreme measures might yield quick results, but they are challenging to sustain. Sustainable biohacking prioritizes practices that you can maintain for the long haul.

- **Incremental Changes:** The concept of "kaizen" or continuous improvement is a hallmark of sustainable biohacking. Focus on making small, incremental changes that add up over time.

- **Preventive Health:** Long-term biohacking extends beyond addressing current health issues. It includes preventive strategies to maintain health and reduce the risk of future problems.

16.3 Leveraging Feedback Loops

A key secret to long-term success in biohacking is leveraging feedback loops. These loops provide data and insights that help you make informed decisions and fine-tune your practices:

- **Biometric Feedback:** Utilize biometric measurements like heart rate variability, blood tests, and sleep data to monitor your health.

- **Self-Reflection**: Regularly review your Progress Tracking Notebook to gain insights into what is working and what requires adjustment.

- **Professional Guidance:** Consult with healthcare professionals or biohacking experts who can provide valuable feedback and guidance.

16.4 Community and Support

Joining a biohacking community or having a support network can significantly contribute to your long-term success. These communities offer:

- **Accountability:** Sharing your goals and progress with others keeps you accountable for your actions.

- **Knowledge Sharing:** Interacting with like-minded individuals allows you to exchange knowledge and learn from their experiences.

- **Motivation:** Being part of a community provides ongoing motivation and encouragement.

16.5 Adaptation and Flexibility

As you integrate biohacking into your life for the long term, you must remain adaptable and flexible. Life circumstances, goals, and health conditions can change, and your biohacking practices may need adjustments.

- **Routine Audits:** Regularly review and audit your biohacking practices to ensure they align with your current goals and circumstances.

- **Be Kind to Yourself**: Be flexible and kind to yourself. Accept that there will be times when you can't follow your routine perfectly, and that's okay.

16.6 Celebrate Milestones

Celebrate your biohacking milestones. Recognize and acknowledge the progress you've made along your journey. Celebrating achievements keeps you motivated and reinforces the positive changes you've implemented.

Biohacking for long-term health and optimal well-being is not just a destination; it's a continuous journey. By integrating biohacking into your lifestyle, maintaining a long-term health perspective, leveraging feedback loops, seeking community and support, and staying adaptable, you can achieve and sustain optimal health and well-being for years to come.

PART VI
References on Nutrition and Exercise

Sample Biohacking Nutrition Regimen: The UltraMind Solution

Author: Dr. Mark Hyman

The UltraMind Solution is a biohacking-inspired nutrition and lifestyle program aimed at optimizing brain health, mental clarity, and overall well-being. It emphasizes the role of nutrition, focusing on whole, unprocessed foods and specific nutrient-rich choices.

Key Principles:

1. Inflammatory Foods Elimination: This regimen encourages the removal of processed foods, sugar, refined grains, and unhealthy fats that contribute to inflammation and cognitive decline.

2. Nutrient-Dense Foods Inclusion: It emphasizes the consumption of foods rich in brain-boosting nutrients such as Omega-3 fatty acids, antioxidants, and vitamins.

3. Balancing Blood Sugar: Maintaining stable blood sugar levels through low-glycemic foods is a key component.

4. Proper Hydration: Staying well-hydrated is essential for brain function and overall health.

5. Intermittent Fasting: Some variations of this regimen incorporate intermittent fasting for improved mental clarity and metabolism.

Sample Meal Plan:

Breakfast: Avocado and salmon omelet with spinach and a side of berries.

Lunch: Grilled chicken salad with mixed greens, walnuts, and olive oil dressing.

Snack: Almonds and dark chocolate.

Dinner: Baked wild-caught salmon with steamed broccoli and quinoa.

Additional Components: The regimen often includes exercise recommendations, stress management techniques, and personalized supplementation based on individual needs.

Results: The UltraMind Solution is designed to enhance cognitive function, mood, and overall health. Individuals who follow this program may experience improved mental clarity, better memory, and reduced risk of cognitive disorders.

Please note that this is a real example of a biohacking-inspired nutrition regimen, authored by Dr. Mark Hyman. It emphasizes the importance of nutrient-dense foods and balancing blood sugar for optimal brain function and overall health.

Sample Biohacking Exercise Regimen: High-Intensity Interval Training (HIIT)

Regimen Overview: High-Intensity Interval Training (HIIT) is a popular biohacking-inspired exercise regimen designed to improve cardiovascular fitness, burn fat, and enhance overall physical performance. It focuses on short, intense bursts of exercise followed by brief recovery periods.

Key Principles:

1. Short, Intense Workouts: HIIT workouts typically last 20-30 minutes and consist of short bursts of intense exercise (e.g., sprints, jump squats, or burpees).

2. Interval Training: HIIT alternates between high-intensity periods (e.g., 20 seconds) and low-intensity or rest periods (e.g., 10 seconds).

3. Variability: To prevent adaptation and maintain effectiveness, the exercises and intervals are varied regularly.

4. Full-Body Engagement: HIIT can incorporate a wide range of exercises, ensuring full-body engagement for strength and cardiovascular improvements.

Sample Workout:

Warm-up: 5 minutes of light jogging or jumping jacks.

Interval 1: 20 seconds of maximum effort sprinting.

Recovery: 10 seconds of walking.

Interval 2: 20 seconds of jump squats.

Recovery: 10 seconds of rest.

Interval 3: 20 seconds of push-ups.

Recovery: 10 seconds of rest.

(Repeat the intervals for about 20-30 minutes.)

Frequency: HIIT workouts can be done 3-4 times a week, allowing adequate time for recovery.

Results: HIIT is known for its efficiency in burning calories, improving cardiovascular health, increasing metabolic rate, and building muscle strength. It's a biohacking exercise regimen often chosen for its time-saving and performance-enhancing benefits.

Please note that this is a real example of a biohacking-inspired exercise regimen, focusing on High-Intensity Interval Training (HIIT). It is designed to optimize fitness and overall physical performance through short, intense workouts with interval training principles.

CONCLUSION

In this comprehensive guide to biohacking, we've explored the fascinating world of optimizing human potential and well-being. From understanding the core principles of biohacking to delving into the intricacies of nutrition, exercise, and mind-body synergy, you've gained valuable insights into how to take control of your health and performance. Biohacking empowers you to be the best version of yourself by implementing personalized, science-based strategies.

Throughout the journey, we've touched on the importance of patience, self-control, and adapting to overcome challenges, ensuring you are well-prepared for the road ahead. We've also introduced you to powerful tools, such as the role of technology, that can enhance your biohacking journey.

As you embark on your biohacking adventure, remember that it's a path of self-discovery and constant improvement. Your personalized biohacking plan will be your guide, allowing you to set clear goals, assess your progress, and stay committed to the journey. Monitoring your results and adapting to changes will be key to your success.

Biohacking is not only about optimizing your health and performance, but it's also about taking charge of your well-being, enhancing your longevity, and achieving your personal goals. It's a journey of empowerment and self-realization, and it's a journey that never truly ends.

Thank You for Choosing This Book

We would like to express our sincere gratitude to you, our readers, for choosing to embark on this biohacking journey with us. Your curiosity, dedication, and commitment to self-improvement are truly commendable.

We hope this book has equipped you with the knowledge and tools you need to take the first steps in your biohacking adventure. Your pursuit of a healthier, more fulfilling life is inspiring. Remember that every small change you make contributes to the greater transformation you seek.

Should you have any questions, seek further guidance, or want to explore specific aspects of biohacking in more detail, the resources, references, and community of biohackers are at your disposal.

As you move forward, may your biohacking journey be filled with success, resilience, and the rewards of optimal health and well-being. Continue to explore, adapt, and always strive for progress. You have the power to redefine your potential, and the future is full of exciting possibilities.

Wishing you all the best on your biohacking adventure!

With gratitude,